Hello healthier you

This edition published by Parragon Books Ltd in 2018

Parragon Books Ltd
Chartist House
15–17 Trim Street
Bath BA1 1HA, UK
www.parragon.com

Written by Frances Prior-Reeves
Illustrated by Julie Mackey
Edited by Hannah Kelly
Designed by Will Offer

ISBN 978-1-4748-6927-0

Printed in China

Note:
While the publisher has made all reasonable efforts to ensure that the information contained
in this book is accurate and up to date at the time of publication, anyone reading this book
should note the following important points:-

Medical and pharmaceutical knowledge is constantly changing and the author and the
publisher cannot and do not guarantee the accuracy or appropriateness of the contents of
this book;
In any event, this book is not intended to be, and should not be relied upon, as a substitute
for appropriate, tailored professional advice. Both the author and the publisher strongly
recommend that a doctor or other healthcare professional is consulted before embarking on
major dietary changes;
For the reasons set out above, and to the fullest extent permitted by law, the author and
publisher: (i) cannot and do not accept any legal duty of care or responsibility in relation
to the accuracy or appropriateness of the contents of this book, even where expressed as
'advice' or using other words to this effect; and (ii) disclaim any liability, loss, damage or risk
that may be claimed or incurred as a consequence – directly or indirectly – of the use and/or
application of any of the contents of this book.

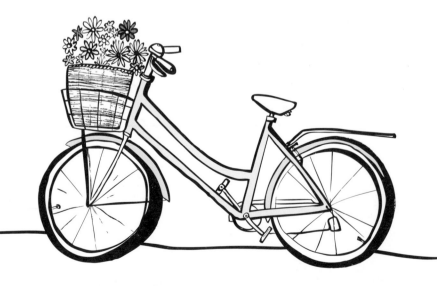

Hello healthier you

A motivational companion to weight loss

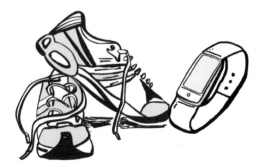

PaRragon

Bath · New York · Cologne · Melbourne · Delhi
Hong Kong · Shenzhen · Singapore

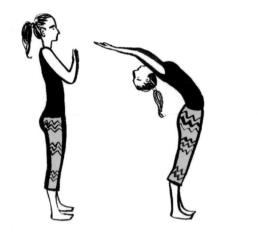
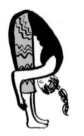
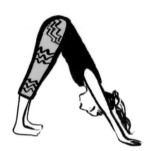

NEW BEGINNINGS

Today is a new beginning and this book is here to guide you to a happier and healthier lifestyle.

Inside these pages you'll find:

- A 30-week diary to log your food and exercise
- Space to track your calorie intake, sleep and active minutes
- Inspiring and motivational tips and quotes to make losing weight easier
- Pages to plan workouts and meals for the week ahead
- Healthy and feel-good recipes
- Plenty of space to reflect on each week and add journal thoughts

Think positive

Just by opening this book you're one step closer to where you want to be. The advice and tips are simple to follow and you can dip in and out of the book anytime you please. Just remember – small changes can make a big impact.

This is your private notebook to transform any negative feelings towards your weight and body into a positive attitude. It is a space where you can be honest, because being honest with yourself is the best way to face up to your challenges and do something to overcome them.

You won't find fad diets here, or ways to force you to abstain from the things you love. But you will find plenty of fun and interesting ideas to help you reach your weight-loss goals.

Celebrate the small but significant triumphs and be happy with any progress you make. Let *Hello Healthier You* teach you how to be kind to yourself and be your essential companion on this weight-loss journey.

Let's get started, there's no time like the present.

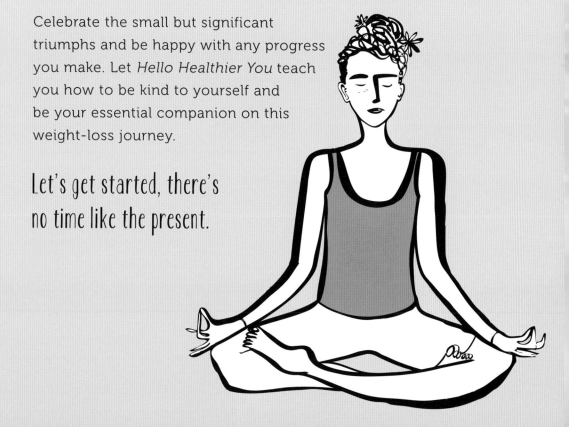

START TODAY!

There's always a reason to put off your start date, but starting today will make you one day closer to the healthier and happier you.

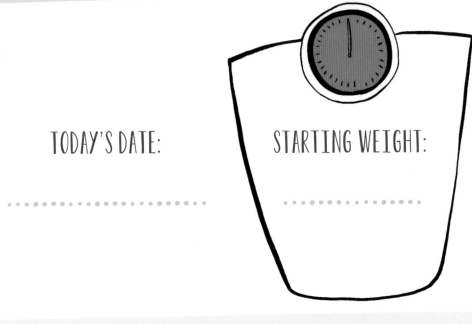

TODAY'S DATE:

. . . .

STARTING WEIGHT:

. . . .

Write a list of personal goals. Don't put a time limit against these goals – it's not a finish line, it's a journey to a new you.

- ....
  ....
- ....
  ....
- ....
  ....

- ....
  ....
- ....
  ....
- ....
  ....

Write a motivational note to yourself that you can look back on over the coming weeks. Include a list of things you want to achieve and the reasons why you're doing this.

To Me,

From Me.

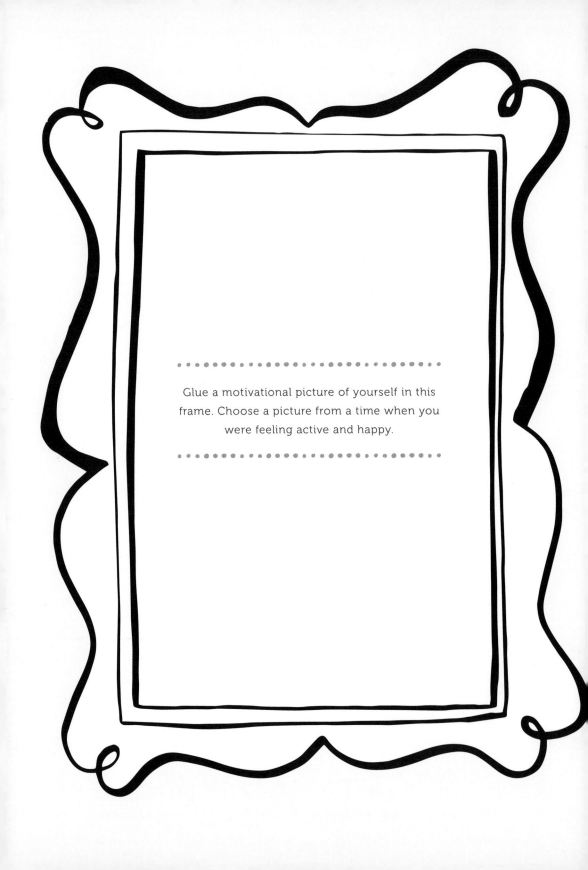

Glue a motivational picture of yourself in this frame. Choose a picture from a time when you were feeling active and happy.

RECORD YOUR MEASUREMENTS

Record your measurements here, at 15 weeks, and then again at the end of the book, but you can measure yourself at any stage along your weight-loss journey.

chest ....

upper arms ....

orearms ....

waist ....

hips ....

thighs ....

calves ....

Measuring yourself is a fantastic way to track your changing body shape as you get fitter. You might find the results more noticeable than weighing yourself.

LOSE WEIGHT BY EATING!

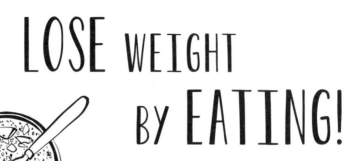

Don't concentrate on what you can't eat or the junk food you'll miss. Use this space to fill in your favourite meals that are 'healthy'.

BREAKFAST

LUNCH

DINNER

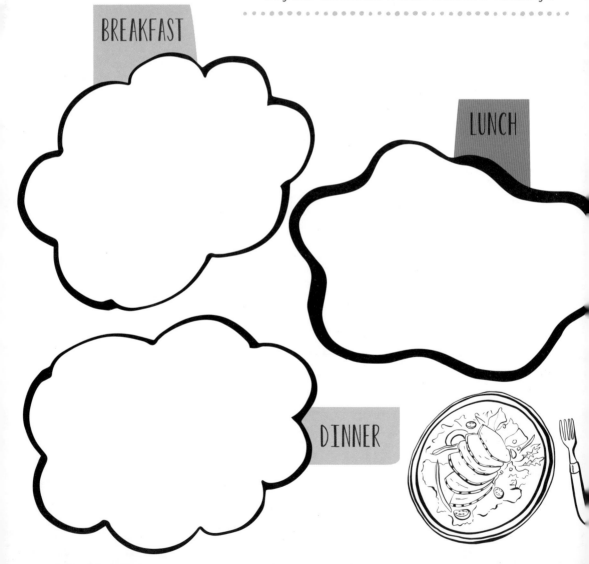

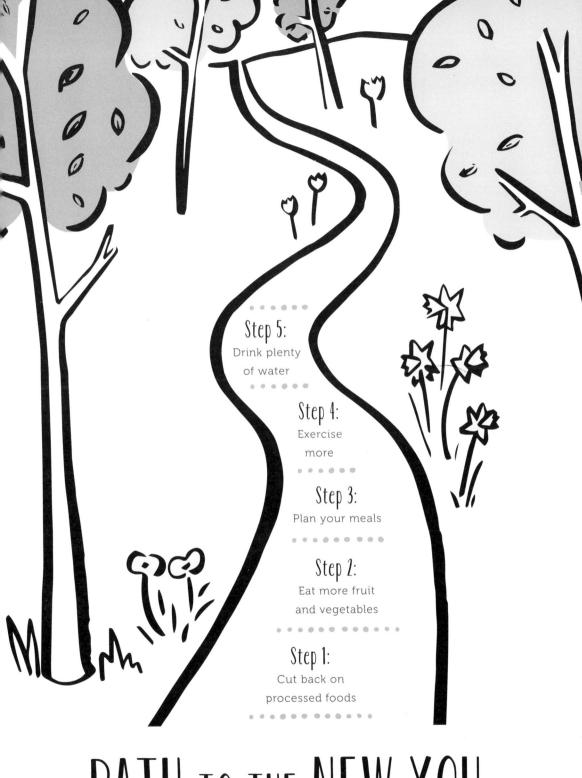

Step 5:
Drink plenty
of water

Step 4:
Exercise
more

Step 3:
Plan your meals

Step 2:
Eat more fruit
and vegetables

Step 1:
Cut back on
processed foods

PATH TO THE NEW YOU

PLAN YOUR MEALS

- Use the space in this book to plan breakfast, lunch and dinner for a week. Then start your own meal calendar so you can plan for the year!

- Planning your meals will save you time and money, as well as keep your diet on track.

- Plan for leftovers and if you don't want it right away freeze it. The meal will taste just as good a week later.

- Cooking for yourself with fresh food is the best way to know exactly what you're consuming and will generally include less sugar and salt.

- Spend time looking for new recipes and save them somewhere that works for you – a scrapbook, online and there's space in this book to record them too.

- Write a shopping list before you go to the shops so you'll be less likely to add unhealthy items to the trolley.

- Don't go to the supermarket with an empty stomach.

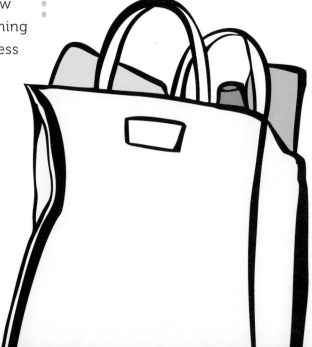

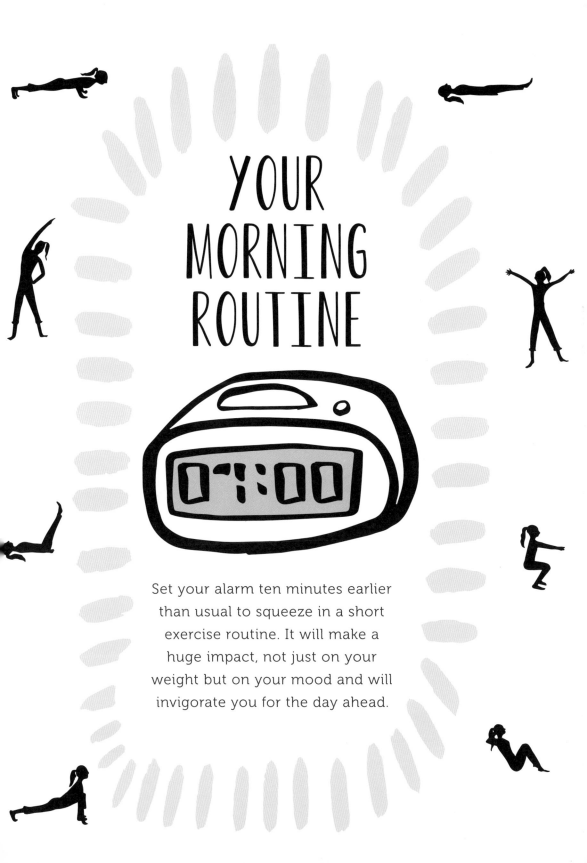

YOUR MORNING ROUTINE

Set your alarm ten minutes earlier than usual to squeeze in a short exercise routine. It will make a huge impact, not just on your weight but on your mood and will invigorate you for the day ahead.

STARTING A
FOOD & EXERCISE DIARY

You don't have to be a gym junkie to become
healthier, you just need to move more.

Throughout the book you will find a weekly diary, covering 30 weeks.
This is space for you to log what you eat and how much exercise you
do each day. Record what you eat for breakfast, lunch, dinner and
the snacks in-between and log the calories consumed.

Start tracking your stats and see how much you actually move. Note
your averages and try to improve on them. You'll see if the amount
you exercise or the hours of sleep you have affect your mood.

You can use an electronic tracker app to record the stats or just keep
note throughout the day. Add the stats to every day of the weekly
diary when you see the icons below:

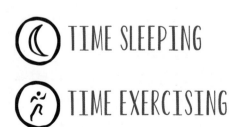 TIME SLEEPING

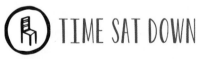 TIME SAT DOWN

TIME EXERCISING

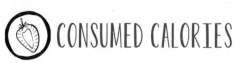 CONSUMED CALORIES

If you're serious about choosing a healthier lifestyle then you need to be completely honest with YOURSELF about what you eat.

NOTE DOWN THE BAD FOOD CHOICES AS WELL AS THE GOOD.

Try to get moving for at least 60 minutes a day, although, you should aim to do enough to raise your heart rate for at least 20 minutes a day.

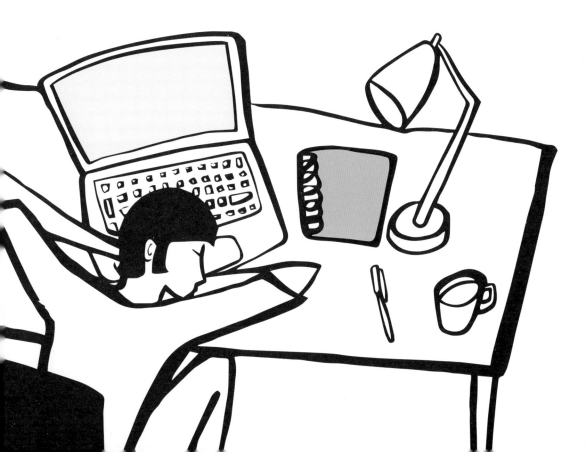

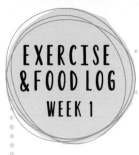

EXERCISE & FOOD LOG
WEEK 1

Monday

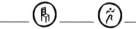

Tuesday

Wednesday

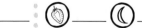

Thursday

🍓 —— 🌙 —— 🪑 —— 🏃 —

Friday

🍓 —— 🌙 —— 🪑 —— 🏃 —

Saturday

🍓 —— 🌙 —— 🪑 —— 🏃 —

Sunday

🍓 —— 🌙 —
🪑 —— 🏃 —

WEIGHT:

. . . .

YOUR GOALS

WHAT ARE YOUR FITNESS GOALS?

....

....

....

....

Write down where you are now and where you'd like to be.

CURRENT		TARGET

.... Weight ....

.... Waist measurement ....

.... Active minutes per day ....

.... Approx. number of steps per day ....

.... Calories per day ....

.... Alcohol units per week ....

.... Number of hours sleep per night ....

Experiment with different forms of exercise to get you motivated. Draw a star next to ones you like.

Kettle bells

Yoga

Pilates

Martial arts

Spinning

Tai Chi

Swimming

Power walking

Badminton

Squash

Tennis

Cycling

Body balance

Aerobics

Dancing

Zumba

Running

Aqua aerobics

Football

Rugby

Weight training

Rock climbing

Throw away all of the bad food hiding in your fridge and at the back of your cupboard – if it's not in your house it can't tempt you.

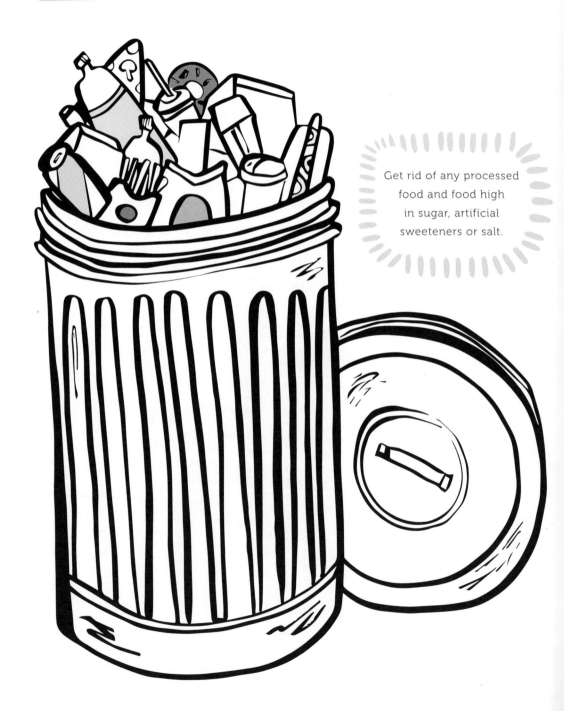

Get rid of any processed food and food high in sugar, artificial sweeteners or salt.

Draw healthy snacks and ingredients that you like in the fridge and cupboard.

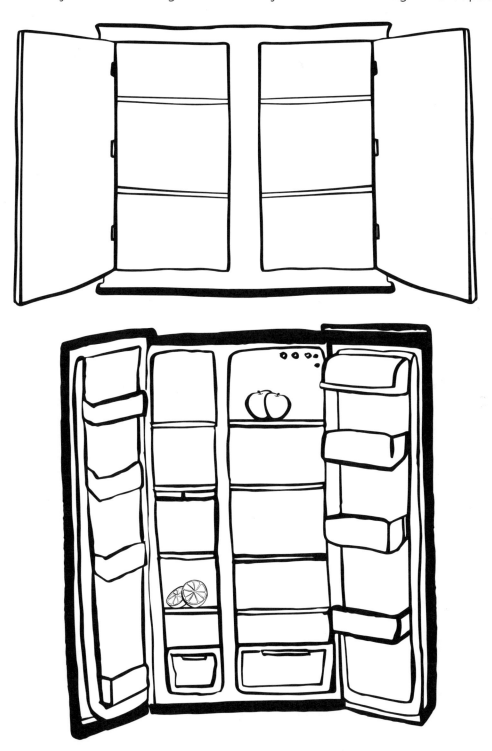

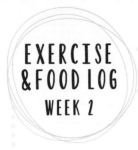

EXERCISE & FOOD LOG
WEEK 2

Monday

———

Tuesday

Wednesday

————

——

Thursday

Friday

🍓 —— ☾ —— 🪑 —— 🏃 ——   🍓 —— ☾ —— 🪑 —— 🏃 ——

Saturday

Sunday

🍓 —— ☾ —— 🪑 —— 🏃 ——   🍓 —— ☾ ——
                                    🪑 —— 🏃 ——

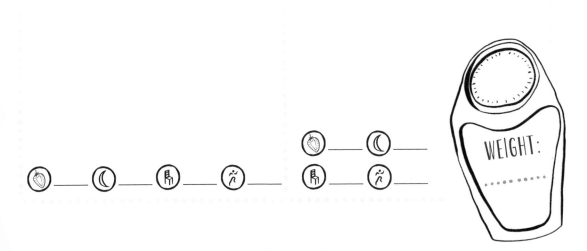

WEIGHT:

. . . .

DRINK PLENTY OF WATER

Water is essential for your body – it aids digestion and avoids dehydration. Guidelines suggest drinking 6–8 glasses (1.2 litres) a day. Make copies of this chart, then colour in a glass every time you drink one to make sure you're drinking enough.

MONDAY

TUESDAY

WEDNESDAY

THURSDAY

FRIDAY

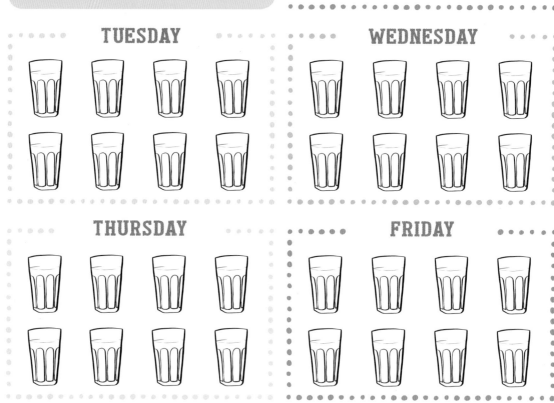

SATURDAY

SUNDAY

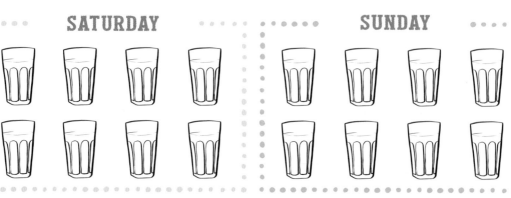

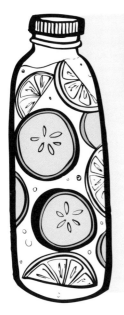

KIWI & CUCUMBER INFUSED WATER

Chilled water is infused with kiwi and cucumber to make this cleansing and refreshing drink. Served with zesty lemon ice cubes, it is a great thirst-quencher, especially when you're feeling hot and tired.

Ingredients

½ cucumber

2 kiwis, peeled and thickly sliced

1 litre/1¾ pints chilled water

Lemon Ice Cubes

zest of 1 lemon

water, to fill an ice-cube tray

Instructions

1. Make your lemon ice cubes at least 4 hours before they are needed. Cut the lemon zest into pieces that will sit neatly in the holes of an ice-cube tray. Place the zest pieces in the holes of the tray and fill the holes with water. Freeze for at least 4–6 hours, or until needed.

2. When ready to serve, peel ribbons from a cucumber using a vegetable peeler. Place the ribbons in the bottom of a jug, along with the fresh kiwi slices.

3. Add the lemon zest ice cubes to the jug and top up with the chilled water. Serve immediately.

Monday

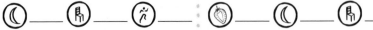

Tuesday

Wednesday

Thursday

🍓 ___ 🌙 ___ 🪑 ___ 🏃 ___

Friday

🍓 ___ 🌙 ___ 🪑 ___ 🏃 ___

Saturday

🍓 ___ 🌙 ___ 🪑 ___ 🏃 ___

Sunday

🍓 ___ 🌙 ___
🪑 ___ 🏃 ___

WEIGHT:

. . . .

TRACKING
YOUR STEPS

It is recommended to walk 10,000 steps each day. This can seem very high but you'll be surprised by how much your steps increase if you try to move around more in between workouts. You can use a pedometer or tracker app to record your steps, but 2,000 steps equate to approximately 1 mile or 15 to 20 minutes of brisk walking.

The best step goal is the one you'll be able to reach and stick with. Aim to be more active today than you were yesterday.

Track your steps for a week either with a pedometer or your total walking time each day.

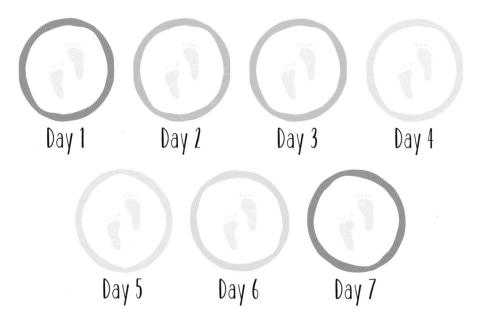

Day 1   Day 2   Day 3   Day 4

Day 5   Day 6   Day 7

To hit your step goal you'll need to create new habits:

- (⚐) Go for a walk with a friend, spouse or child.

- (⚐) Get off the bus early.

- (⚐) Walk to speak to a colleague rather than emailing them.

- (⚐) Take the stairs rather than the lift.

- (⚐) Set a reminder every hour to do a lap of the building or block.

- (⚐) Don't try and force all of your steps into one long walk – make time for three 30-minute brisk walks a day.

- (⚐) Every time you make a phone call pace around or take your call outside on a mobile phone.

- (⚐) Park in the furthest corner of the car park.

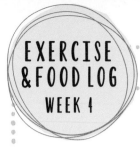

EXERCISE & FOOD LOG
WEEK 4

Monday

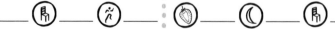

Tuesday

Wednesday

 — — — —

 —  — — —

Thursday

🍓 ___ ☾ ___ 🪑 ___ 🏃 ___

Friday

🍓 ___ ☾ ___ 🪑 ___ 🏃 ___

Saturday

🍓 ___ ☾ ___ 🪑 ___ 🏃 ___

Sunday

🍓 ___ ☾ ___
🪑 ___ 🏃 ___

WEIGHT:

Mindfulness is a way to focus on your feelings, thoughts and body, while in the present moment, in order to create a sense of awareness and calm.

Mindful eating helps you to eat at a slower pace, savour all of the flavours of what you're eating and enjoy every mouthful.

Challenge

Try and eat mindfully for every meal this week and pay attention to what you're consuming. Make note of the smells, the flavours, and your thoughts and feelings while you eat.

Have you ever been watching a film and ten minutes into it realized that the box of popcorn in front of you has already gone?

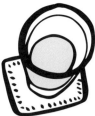

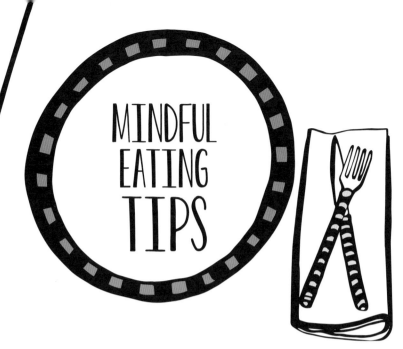

MINDFUL EATING TIPS

- Never eat straight from the fridge or cupboard – put your food on a plate.

- Take one bite at a time. Don't start the next until your mouth is completely empty.

- Cook and eat in a good mood. Don't eat when you're feeling emotional.

- Stop eating when you're feeling full, not when your plate is empty.

- Don't multitask whilst eating. These distractions could make you eat more.

- Don't hurry. Try playing some relaxing music to open up another sense.

- Don't clear your plate out of politeness but equally don't only eat one bite because people are watching.

- Savour the different flavours. Pretend you're a food critic.

- Drink plenty of water throughout the meal.

- Research portion sizes. You'll be pleasantly surprised at the size of your guilt-free portion.

THE MOST IMPORTANT MEAL OF THE DAY

It's important not to skip breakfast, it gives you the energy that you need for the day ahead. You should leave the house feeling full – make time for a mindful breakfast.

Blitz frozen berries with protein-boosting cashew and Brazil nuts, porridge oats and almond milk for a healthy breakfast smoothie.

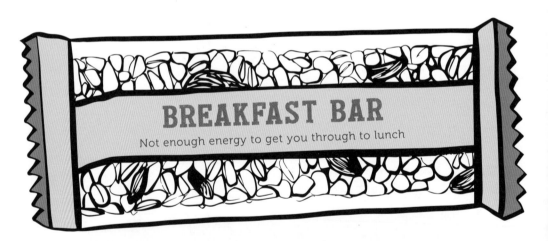

BREAKFAST BAR

Not enough energy to get you through to lunch

Be kind to yourself and feed your body the nutrients it needs for the day.

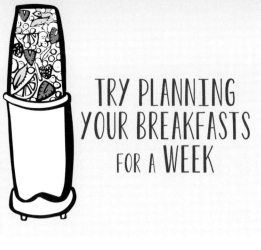

TRY PLANNING YOUR BREAKFASTS FOR A WEEK

MONDAY

TUESDAY

WEDNESDAY

THURSDAY

FRIDAY

SATURDAY

SUNDAY

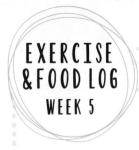

EXERCISE & FOOD LOG
WEEK 5

Monday

 —— —— —— ——

Tuesday

Wednesday

 —— —— —— ——

 —— —— —— ——

Thursday

🍓 ___ ☾ ___ 🪑 ___ 🏃 ___

Friday

🍓 ___ ☾ ___ 🪑 ___ 🏃 ___

Saturday

🍓 ___ ☾ ___ 🪑 ___ 🏃 ___

Sunday

🍓 ___ ☾ ___
🪑 ___ 🏃 ___

WEIGHT:

. . . .

WEEK 5 REFLECTION

Use this space to reflect on your first five weeks. Add doodles, progress graphs, lists, mood charts. Release your creativity.

IT'S NOT ALL ABOUT WEIGHT LOSS!

Be mindful of everything in your life. Healthy eating needs to be done in line with other lifestyle changes.

HEALTHY EATING

GOOD SLEEP

HEALTHY LIFE

STRESS MANAGEMENT

REGULAR EXERCISE

PLENTY OF WATER

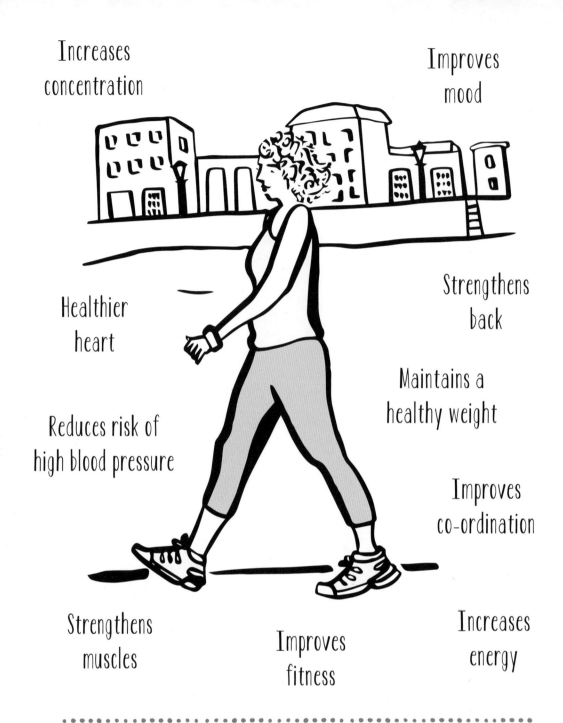

BENEFITS of WALKING

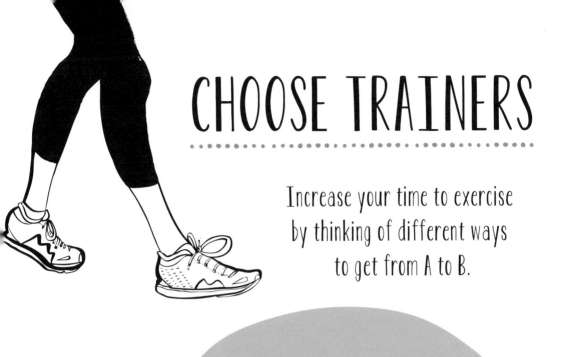

CHOOSE TRAINERS

Increase your time to exercise
by thinking of different ways
to get from A to B.

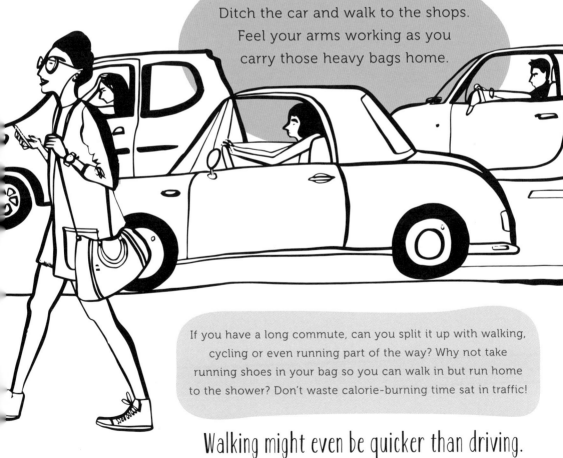

Ditch the car and walk to the shops.
Feel your arms working as you
carry those heavy bags home.

If you have a long commute, can you split it up with walking,
cycling or even running part of the way? Why not take
running shoes in your bag so you can walk in but run home
to the shower? Don't waste calorie-burning time sat in traffic!

Walking might even be quicker than driving.

EXERCISE & FOOD LOG
WEEK 6

Monday

Tuesday

Wednesday

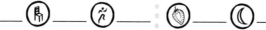

Thursday

Friday

🍓 ⬤ —— 🌙 ⬤ —— 🪑 ⬤ —— 🏃 ⬤ ——   🍓 ⬤ —— 🌙 ⬤ —— 🪑 ⬤ —— 🏃 ⬤ ——

Saturday

Sunday

🍓 ⬤ —— 🌙 ⬤ —— 🪑 ⬤ —— 🏃 ⬤ ——   🍓 ⬤ —— 🌙 ⬤ ——

🪑 ⬤ —— 🏃 ⬤ ——

WEIGHT:

. . . .

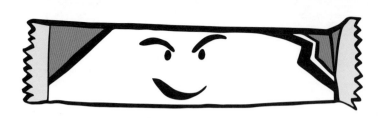

FEED
YOUR BODY
NOT YOUR
EMOTIONS

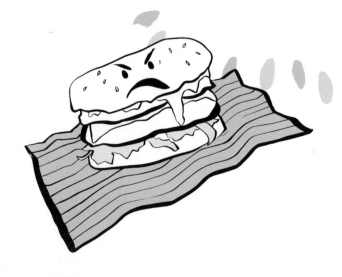

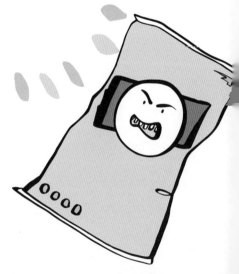

Write a list of things you know trigger emotional eating:

Can you resolve or avoid any of these situations? Give your
mind time to come to terms with things.

Monday

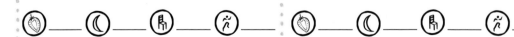

Tuesday

Wednesday

Thursday

🍓 —— 🌙 —— 🪑 —— 🏃 ——

Friday

🍓 —— 🌙 —— 🪑 —— 🏃 ——

Saturday

🍓 —— 🌙 —— 🪑 —— 🏃 ——

Sunday

🍓 —— 🌙 ——

🪑 —— 🏃 ——

WEIGHT:

. . . .

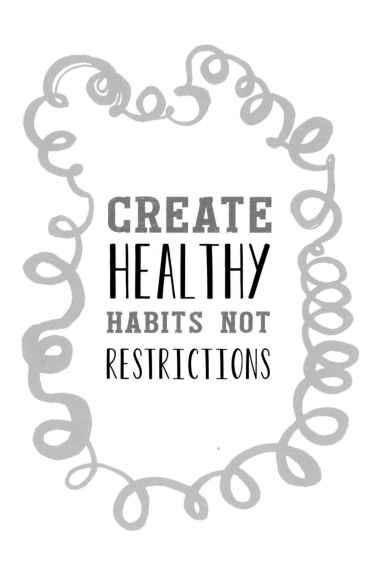

CREATE
HEALTHY
HABITS NOT
RESTRICTIONS

LEGS UP THE WALL

This is a great daily restorative exercise you could do before bed, and it only takes five minutes. It's supportive for your nervous system and digestion, reduces fatigue in your legs, and can lower your heart rate.

Concentrating on your breathing will help you cultivate a quiet mind, calm the stresses of the day and rejuvenate you.

1. Make sure your bottom is in contact with the wall, getting close can be tricky but it'll get easier.

2. Place your arms by your side, close your eyes, clear your mind and concentrate on your breathing.

3. Stay here for five minutes. If you have lower back problems, a bolster underneath your bottom may help.

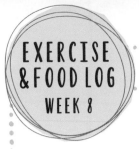

EXERCISE & FOOD LOG
WEEK 8

Monday

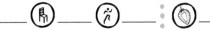

Tuesday

Wednesday

Thursday

🍓◯—☾◯—🪑◯—🏃◯—

Friday

🍓◯—☾◯—🪑◯—🏃◯—

Saturday

🍓◯—☾◯—🪑◯—🏃◯—

Sunday

🍓◯—☾◯
🪑◯—🏃◯

WEIGHT:

Don't remove fun from your life when you ditch the calories. Dieting doesn't have to be dull.

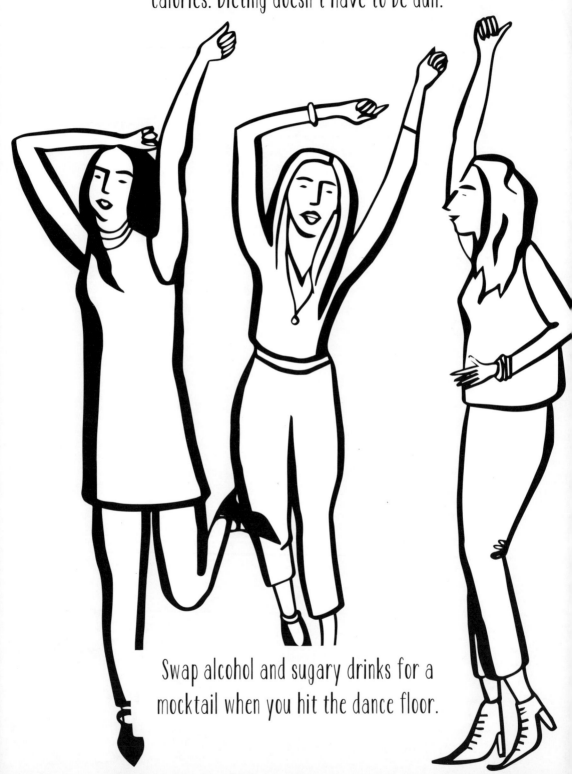

Swap alcohol and sugary drinks for a mocktail when you hit the dance floor.

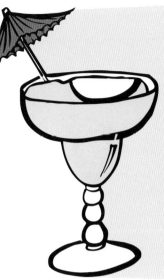

MELON & COCONUT
MOCK MOJITO

This vivid green mock mojito is loaded with nourishing nutrients and can be whizzed up in minutes, providing an essential energy boost before hitting the dance floor. Make a jug of this mocktail to share with friends.

Ingredients

20 g/¾ oz spinach

50 g/1¾ oz coconut flesh

200 ml/7 fl oz chilled water

100 g/3½ oz cantaloupe melon, peeled, deseeded and chopped

1 tbsp chopped fresh mint

juice of ½ lime

50 g/1¾ oz mango, peeled, stoned and chopped, plus 1 extra slice to decorate

crushed ice, to serve, optional

Instructions

1. Place the spinach, coconut and water in a blender and whizz until smooth.

2. Add the melon, mint, lime juice and mango, and blend until smooth and creamy.

3. Pour over crushed ice, if using, and serve immediately, decorated with a mango slice.

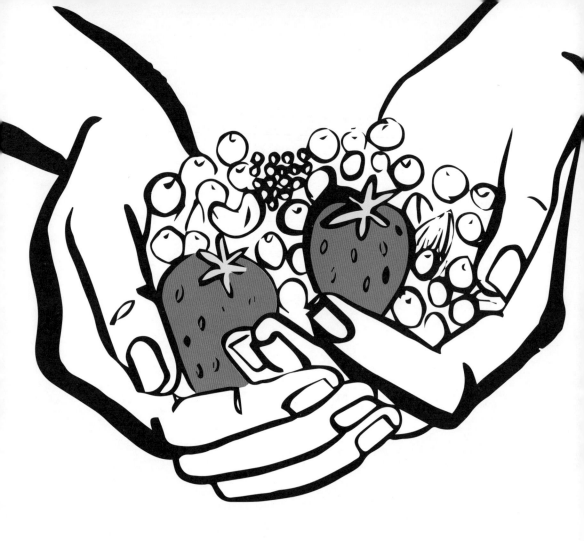

EAT BETTER, NOT LESS!

Healthy snacks are important because we need to keep fuelled between meals, but make yourself move for them. Don't store snacks in your desk drawer!

CREATE A MANTRA

Make it uplifting! Write it here, repeat it, say it as soon as you wake up, stick a copy to your mirror and recite it when necessary.

I am in charge
of how
I feel

It is enough
to do my
best

I have the
power to create
change

I can
& I will

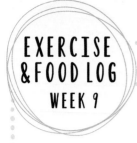

EXERCISE & FOOD LOG
WEEK 9

Monday

 —— —— —— ——

Tuesday

Wednesday

 —— —— —— ——

 —— —— —— ——

Thursday

Friday

🍓 —— 🌙 —— 🪑 —— 🏃 —— 🍓 —— 🌙 —— 🪑 —— 🏃 ——

Saturday

Sunday

🍓 —— 🌙 —— 🪑 —— 🏃 ——

🍓 —— 🌙 ——
🪑 —— 🏃 ——

WEIGHT:

· · · · · · · ·

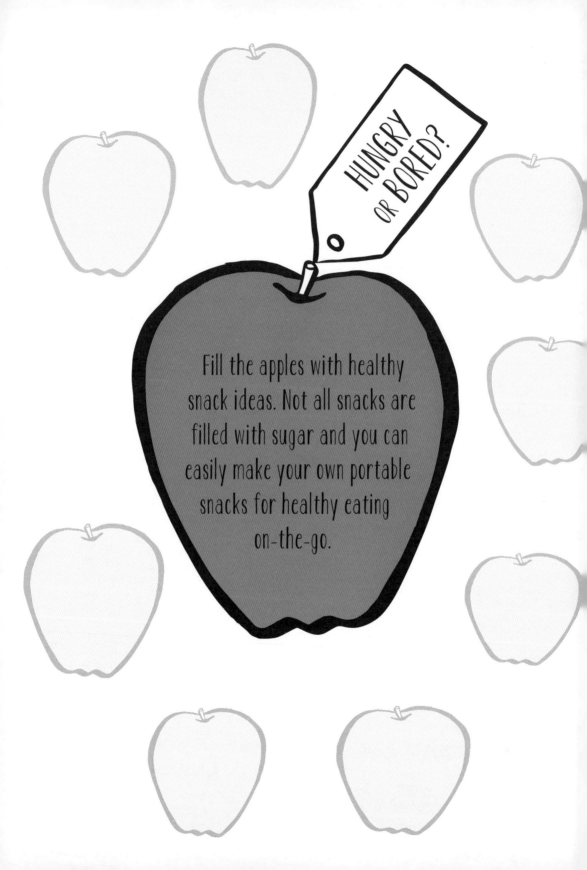

HUNGRY OR BORED?

Fill the apples with healthy snack ideas. Not all snacks are filled with sugar and you can easily make your own portable snacks for healthy eating on-the-go.

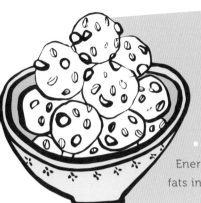

CHOCOLATE & PEANUT BUTTER ENERGY BALLS

Energy balls typically combine protein, carbohydrates and fats in a handy, portable shape.

Ingredients

50 g/1¾ oz blanched almonds

50 g/2¼ oz unsweetened peanut butter

20 g/¾ oz unsalted peanuts, roughly chopped

3 tbsp flaxseeds

30 g/1 oz plain chocolate with 85% cocoa, finely chopped

1 tsp cocoa powder

sea salt (optional)

Instructions

1. Put the blanched almonds in a food processor and process for a minute, until you have the texture of rough flour.

2. Put the peanut butter, peanuts, flaxseeds, chocolate and a small pinch of salt, if using, in a bowl and mix. Add the almond flour, reserving 1½ tablespoons. Mix until you have a texture resembling chunky clay.

3. Sprinkle the remaining almond flour and the cocoa powder onto a plate and mix with a teaspoon. Form a tablespoon-sized blob of the peanut mixture into a ball using your palms. Roll it in the cocoa powder mixture, then transfer to a plate. Make a further seven balls in the same way.

4. Cover and chill in the refrigerator for at least 30 minutes. Store for up to two days.

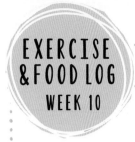
Monday

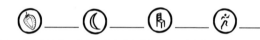

Tuesday

Wednesday

    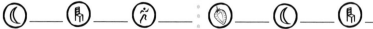

Thursday

Friday

Saturday

Sunday

WEIGHT:

. . . .

CONGRATULATIONS FOR REACHING TEN WEEKS!

Your body will be used to moving more so adding in an extra ten-minute stretch in the morning can be really beneficial for your muscles as well as gearing yourself up for the challenges of the day ahead.

Make up your own routine or follow this simple one, making the movements flow into one another.

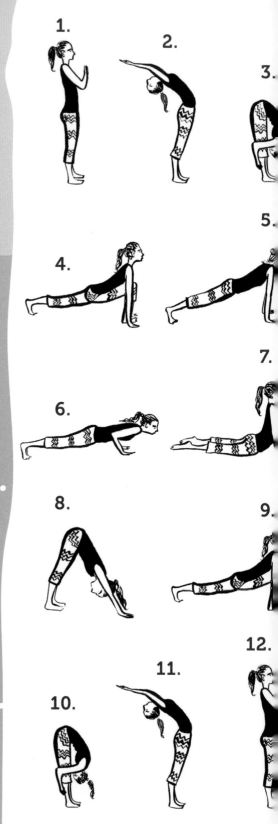

WEEK 10 REFLECTION

Use this space to reflect on the past five weeks. Add doodles, progress graphs, lists, mood charts. Release your creativity.

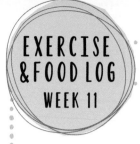

EXERCISE & FOOD LOG
WEEK 11

Monday

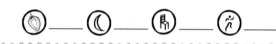

Tuesday

Wednesday

 — — —

 — 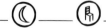 —

Thursday

🍓 __ 🌙 __ 🪑 __ 🏃 __

Friday

🍓 __ 🌙 __ 🪑 __ 🏃 __

Saturday

🍓 __ 🌙 __ 🪑 __ 🏃 __

Sunday

🍓 __ 🌙 __
🪑 __ 🏃 __

WEIGHT:

. . . .

Make lunch the night before so you don't have to rush in the morning. You'll be more likely to make something healthy.

Invest in a lunchbox or bag system that keeps lunches tasting fresh and crisp when you come to eat it later in the day.

Reinvent leftovers from dinner to create fun lunches.

Homemade soup can be quick and inexpensive to make, and extra portions can be frozen for an easy lunch.

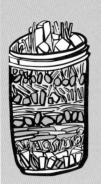

TRY PLANNING YOUR LUNCHES FOR A WEEK

MONDAY

TUESDAY

WEDNESDAY

THURSDAY

FRIDAY

SATURDAY

SUNDAY

MELON BREEZE SOUP

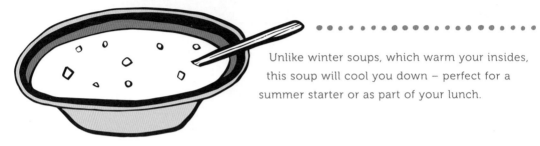

Unlike winter soups, which warm your insides, this soup will cool you down – perfect for a summer starter or as part of your lunch.

Ingredients

300 g/10½ oz green melon, peeled and deseeded

250 g/9 oz cucumber

4 tbsp chopped fresh mint

200 ml/7 fl oz chilled coconut water

1 sprig of fresh mint, to garnish

Instructions

1. Chop the melon and cucumber and place in a blender.

2. Add the mint, pour over the coconut water and blend until smooth and creamy.

3. Serve immediately or chill in the refrigerator and stir just before serving. Garnish with a sprig of mint.

Sleep is a crucial component for a healthy lifestyle.
It can reduce stress and improve your metabolism.

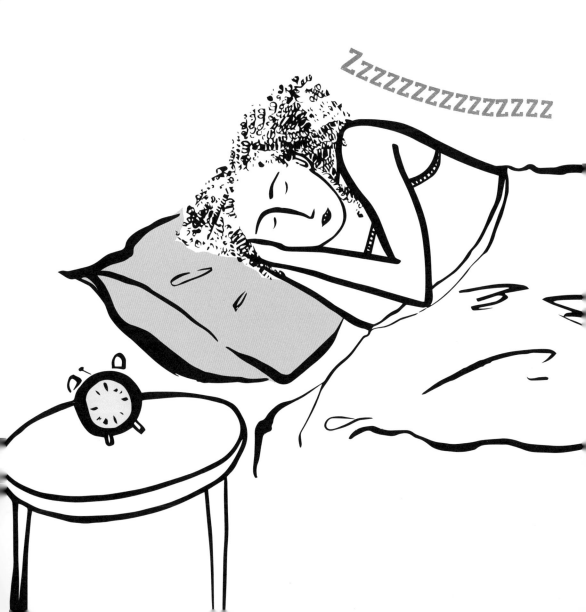

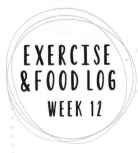

EXERCISE & FOOD LOG
WEEK 12

Monday

 —— —— —— ——

Tuesday

Wednesday

 —— —— —— ——

 —— —— —— ——

Thursday

🍓 ___ 🌙 ___ 🪑 ___ 🏃 ___

Friday

🍓 ___ 🌙 ___ 🪑 ___ 🏃 ___

Saturday

🍓 ___ 🌙 ___ 🪑 ___ 🏃 ___

Sunday

🍓 ___ 🌙 ___

🪑 ___ 🏃 ___

WEIGHT:

. . . .

LET EXERCISE BE YOUR STRESS RELIEVER, NOT FOOD

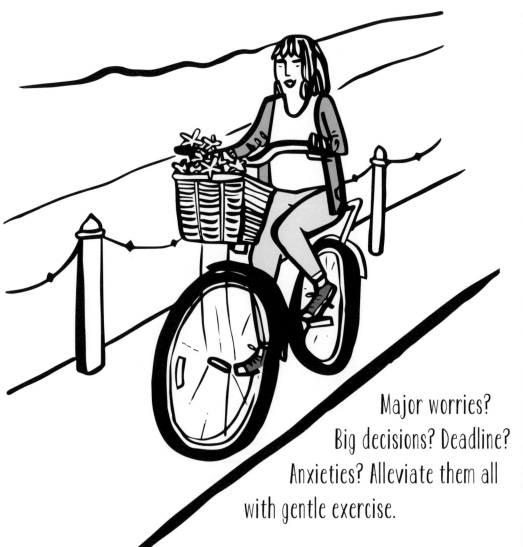

Major worries?
Big decisions? Deadline?
Anxieties? Alleviate them all
with gentle exercise.

It's proven that a little exercise and fresh air will awaken the brain. So, ten minutes outside might help you solve the problem you've been working on for an hour. Time well spent.

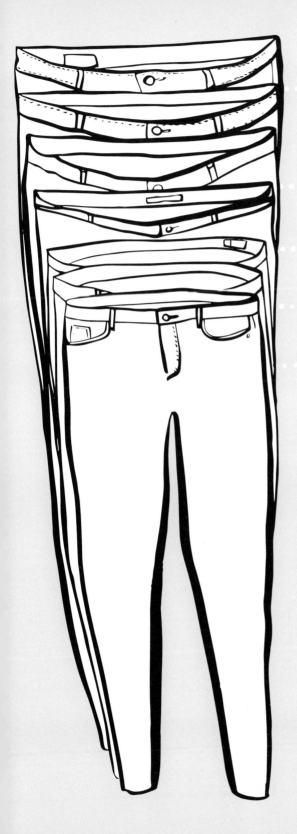

How do I do this?

Slow progress is better than no progress

Look how far I've come already

I can do this!

Yes, I did it!

Colour in the jeans each time you notice some progress, no matter how small it is.

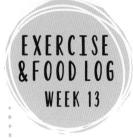

Monday

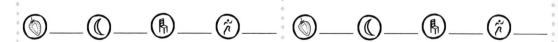

Tuesday

Wednesday

Thursday

🍓___ ☾___ 🪑___ 🏃___

Friday

🍓___ ☾___ 🪑___ 🏃___

Saturday

🍓___ ☾___ 🪑___ 🏃___

Sunday

🍓___ ☾___
🪑___ 🏃___

WEIGHT:

......

THINK OF 10 POSITIVE THINGS

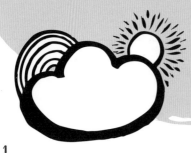

about yourself and
list them below

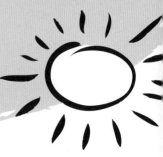

1.
....

2.
....

3.
....

4.
....

5.
....

6.
....

7.
....

8.
....

9.
....

10.
....

Funny **Kind** Hard working **Talented** Intelligent

Always smiling Generous Beautiful **Determine**

fall in love with taking care of yourself

Mind

Spirit   Body

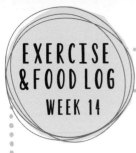

EXERCISE & FOOD LOG
WEEK 14

Monday

 —— —— —— ——

Tuesday

Wednesday

 —— —— —— ——

 —— —— —— ——

Thursday

🍓___ 🌙___ 🪑___ 🏃___

Friday

🍓___ 🌙___ 🪑___ 🏃___

Saturday

🍓___ 🌙___ 🪑___ 🏃___

Sunday

🍓___ 🌙___

🪑___ 🏃___

WEIGHT:

. . . .

Add some tasty, yet healthy, recipes here.

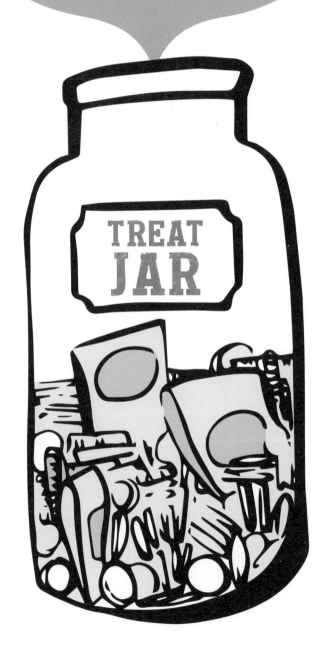

You already know what happens when you give up ...

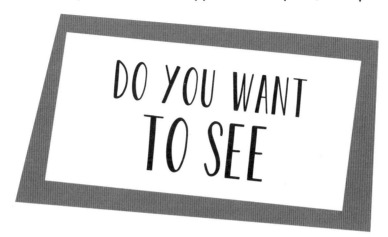

DO YOU WANT
TO SEE

WHAT HAPPENS WHEN

YOU DON'T?

When you feel like giving up, think about why you started. Look back at how far you've come and add any new reasons not to give up.

....

....

....

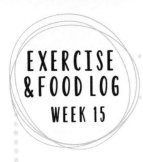

EXERCISE & FOOD LOG
WEEK 15

Monday

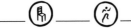

Tuesday

Wednesday

Thursday

Friday

🍓 ── 🌙 ── 🪑 ── 🏃 ──

🍓 ── 🌙 ── 🪑 ── 🏃 ──

Saturday

Sunday

🍓 ── 🌙 ── 🪑 ── 🏃 ──

🍓 ── 🌙 ──
🪑 ── 🏃 ──

WEIGHT:

. . . .

A RECORD of WHERE YOU ARE AT 15 WEEKS

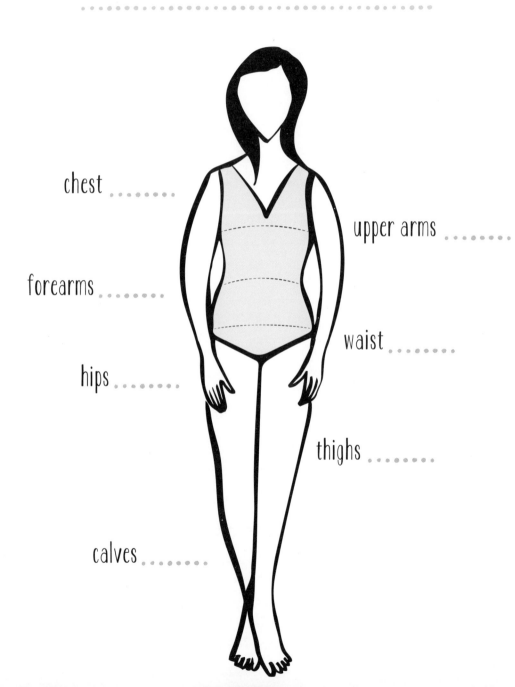

chest ....

upper arms ....

forearms ....

waist ....

hips ....

thighs ....

calves ....

WEEK 15 REFLECTION

Use this space to reflect on the past five weeks. Add doodles, progress graphs, lists, mood charts. Release your creativity.

MUSCLE vs FAT

Adding weights into your exercise routine will help build muscle. Muscle is the same weight as fat but half the size, so it's important to measure as well as weigh yourself.

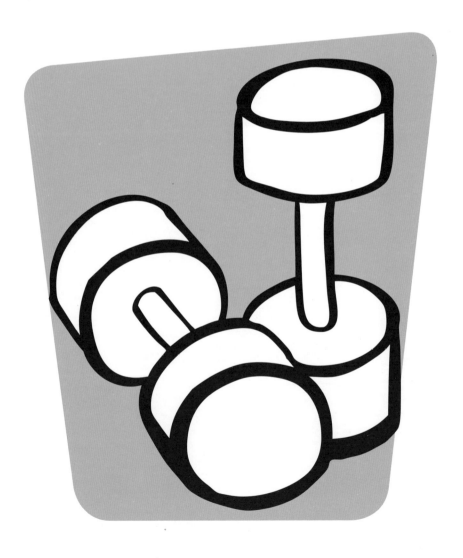

Fill this sun with everything you're
thankful for in your life.

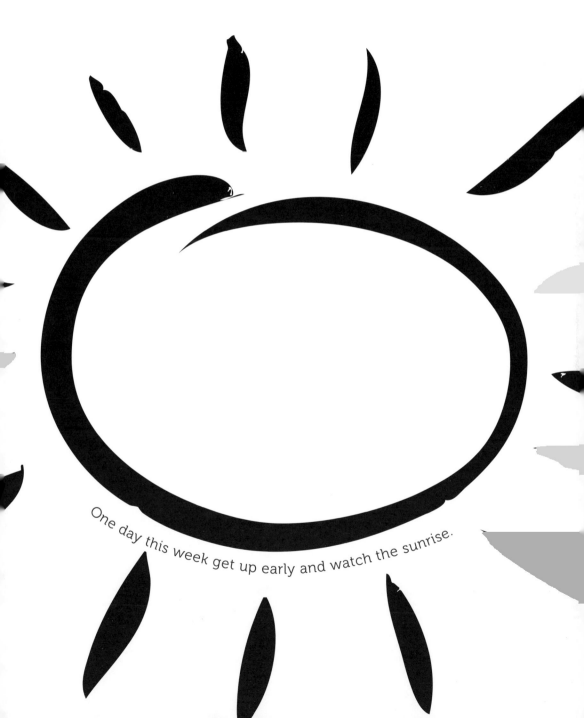

One day this week get up early and watch the sunrise.

Monday

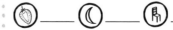

Tuesday

Wednesday

Thursday

🍓 ◯ —— 🌙 ◯ —— 🪑 ◯ —— 🏃 ◯ ——

Friday

🍓 ◯ —— 🌙 ◯ —— 🪑 ◯ —— 🏃 ◯ ——

Saturday

🍓 ◯ —— 🌙 ◯ —— 🪑 ◯ —— 🏃 ◯ ——

Sunday

🍓 ◯ —— 🌙 ◯ ——

🪑 ◯ —— 🏃 ◯ ——

WEIGHT:

· · · · · · · · ·

Your plate should be half full of vegetables or salad, a quarter of healthy protein and a quarter of wholegrains.

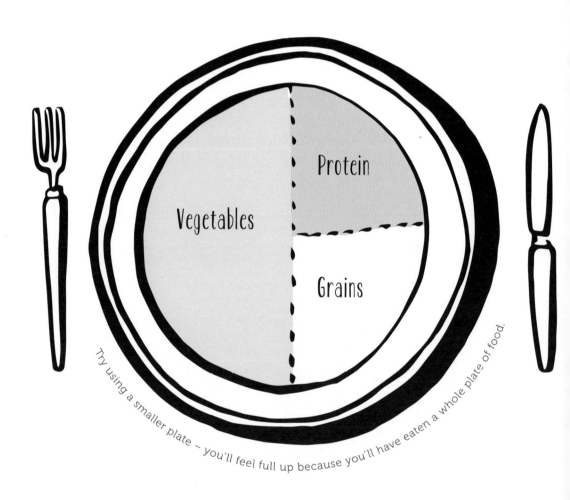

Vegetables

Protein

Grains

Try using a smaller plate – you'll feel full up because you'll have eaten a whole plate of food.

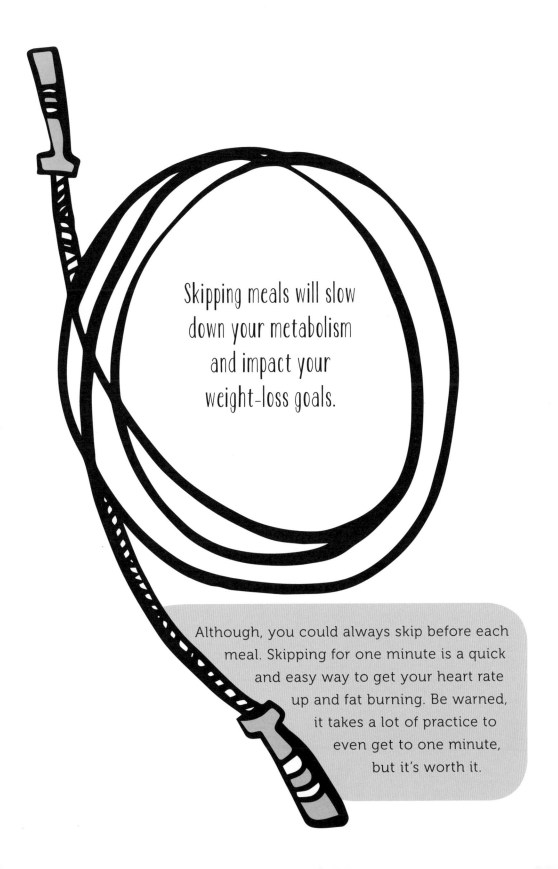

Skipping meals will slow down your metabolism and impact your weight-loss goals.

Although, you could always skip before each meal. Skipping for one minute is a quick and easy way to get your heart rate up and fat burning. Be warned, it takes a lot of practice to even get to one minute, but it's worth it.

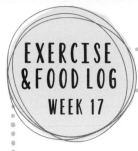

EXERCISE & FOOD LOG
WEEK 17

Monday

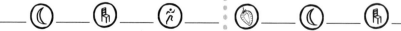

Tuesday

Wednesday

Thursday

🍓◯ —— ☽◯ —— 🪑◯ —— 🏃◯ ——

Friday

🍓◯ —— ☽◯ —— 🪑◯ —— 🏃◯ ——

Saturday

🍓◯ —— ☽◯ —— 🪑◯ —— 🏃◯ ——

Sunday

🍓◯ —— ☽◯ ——
🪑◯ —— 🏃◯ ——

WEIGHT:
....

'Our greatest weakness lies in giving up. The most certain way to success is always to try just one more time.'

THOMAS EDISON

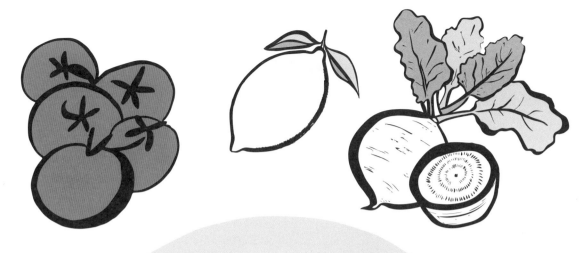

CHALLENGE

Try a week of clean eating – eating
whole foods in their most natural state.
Look for local sources if possible, you'll be
able to find seasonal and nutrient-dense
foods you might otherwise pass over.
Make sure if you eat meat, you try to
include some vegetarian meals.

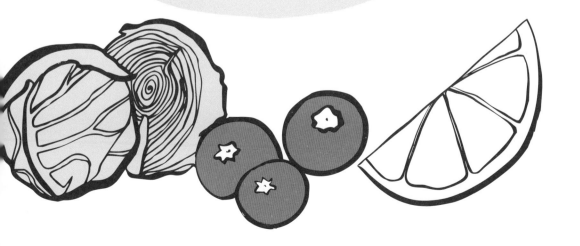

EXERCISE & FOOD LOG
WEEK 18

Monday

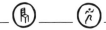

Tuesday

Wednesday

Thursday

🍓 —— 🌙 —— 🪑 —— 🏃 ——

Friday

🍓 —— 🌙 —— 🪑 —— 🏃 ——

Saturday

🍓 —— 🌙 —— 🪑 —— 🏃 ——

Sunday

🍓 —— 🌙 ——

🪑 —— 🏃 ——

WEIGHT:

. . . .

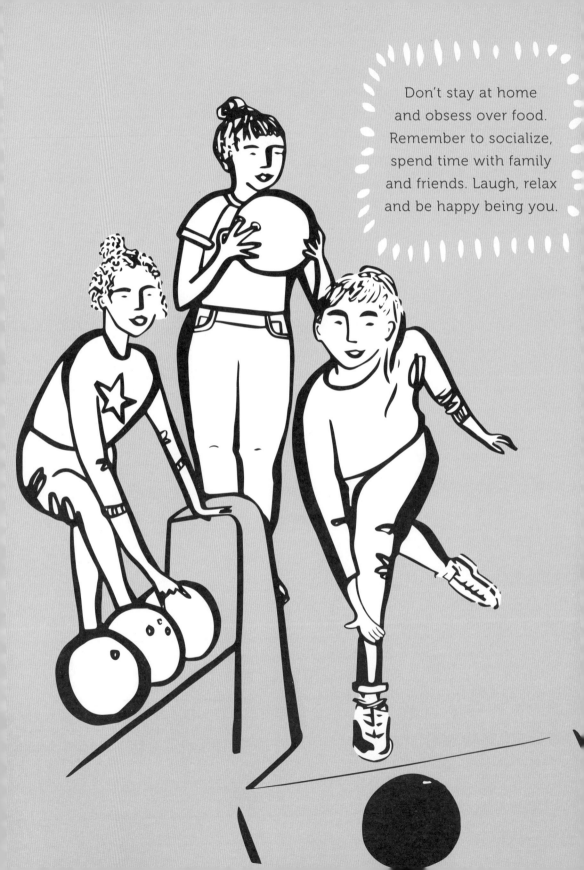

Don't stay at home
and obsess over food.
Remember to socialize,
spend time with family
and friends. Laugh, relax
and be happy being you.

....

....

Theatre

Bowling

Join a book club

....

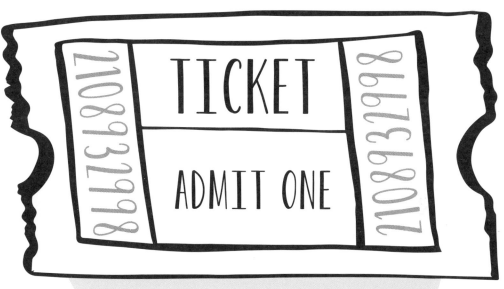

List some activities that aren't food orientated.

Go to a spa

DIY

....

Go to a gig

....

Hiking

....

....

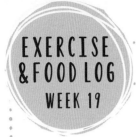

EXERCISE & FOOD LOG
WEEK 19

Monday

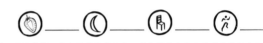

Tuesday

Wednesday

    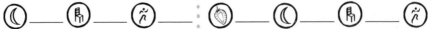

Thursday

🍓___ ☾___ 🪑___ 🏃___

Friday

🍓___ ☾___ 🪑___ 🏃___

Saturday

🍓___ ☾___ 🪑___ 🏃___

Sunday

🍓___ ☾___

🪑___ 🏃___

WEIGHT:

. . . .

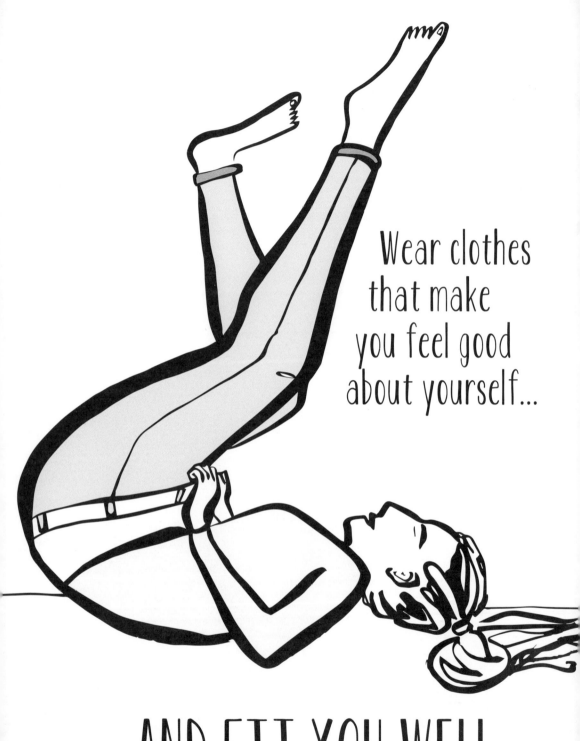

Wear clothes
that make
you feel good
about yourself...

...AND FIT YOU WELL.

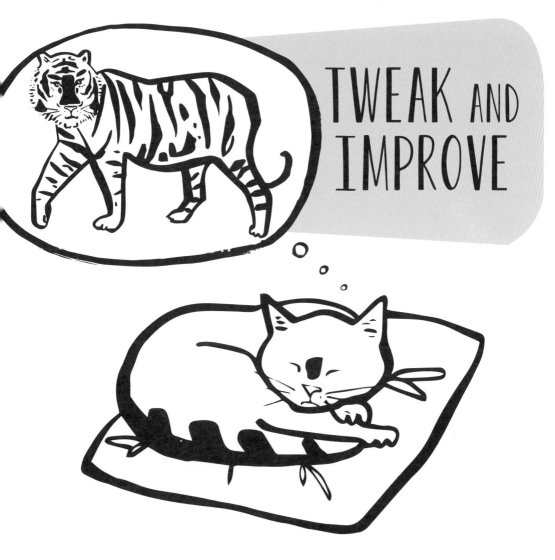

TWEAK AND IMPROVE

Track and adjust your food, exercise, sleep and water intake so that you start to feel healthier and more energetic. Don't just track and hope for different results. If you change your habits and your mindset, your body will soon follow. If it's not working try something new. What small thing can you change to help?

....

....

....

....

HOW ARE YOU?

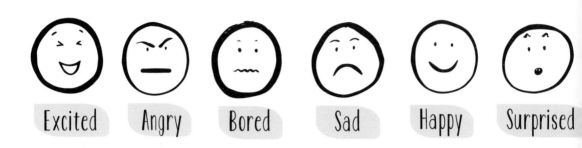

Excited **Angry** **Bored** **Sad** **Happy** **Surprised**

It's a question we're asked all the time but we're not always honest when we reply. Notice how you're feeling each day for a week by completing these emoticons. Do you notice a pattern between your mood, what you're eating and how much you're exercising?

	Morning	Afternoon	Evening
Day 1	◯	◯	◯
Day 2	◯	◯	◯
Day 3	◯	◯	◯
Day 4	◯	◯	◯
Day 5	◯	◯	◯
Day 6	◯	◯	◯
Day 7	◯	◯	◯

Giving up everything that's bad for you will be impossible, so you need to find the right balance.

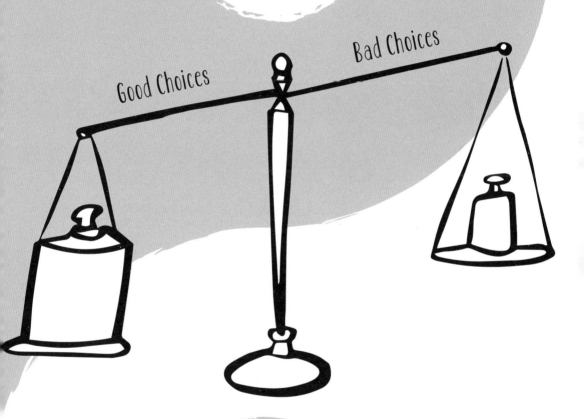

Good Choices

Bad Choices

But, if things aren't changing, you need to alter the balance.

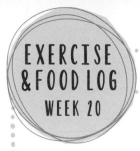

EXERCISE & FOOD LOG
WEEK 20

Monday

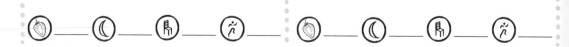

Tuesday

Wednesday

Thursday

🍓 __ 🌙 __ 🪑 __ 🏃 __

Friday

🍓 __ 🌙 __ 🪑 __ 🏃 __

Saturday

🍓 __ 🌙 __ 🪑 __ 🏃 __

Sunday

🍓 __ 🌙 __

🪑 __ 🏃 __

WEIGHT:

. . . .

WEEK 20 REFLECTION

Use this space to reflect on the past five weeks. Add doodles, progress graphs, lists, mood charts. Release your creativity.

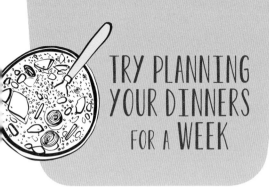

TRY PLANNING YOUR DINNERS FOR A WEEK

MONDAY

TUESDAY

WEDNESDAY

THURSDAY

FRIDAY

SATURDAY

SUNDAY

NO TIME FOR MINDFUL EATING?
DINE AL FRESCO

Move your dinner outdoors to nourish your senses with sights, sounds and smells of nature. You'll be fully engaged in the moment to help you slow down and savour a smaller yet more satisfying portion.

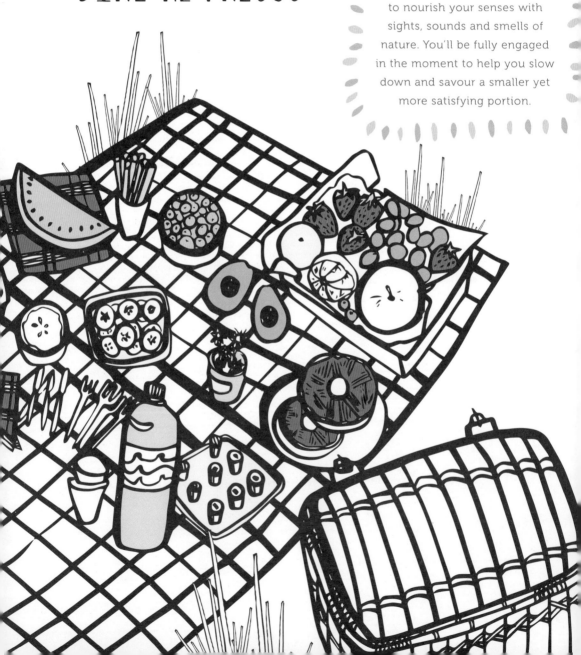

Find an exercise buddy
of a similar stamina,
or someone that's
willing to exercise
at your pace.

We're not all made
for team sports but a
supportive friend will make
exercise enjoyable and help
to motivate you.

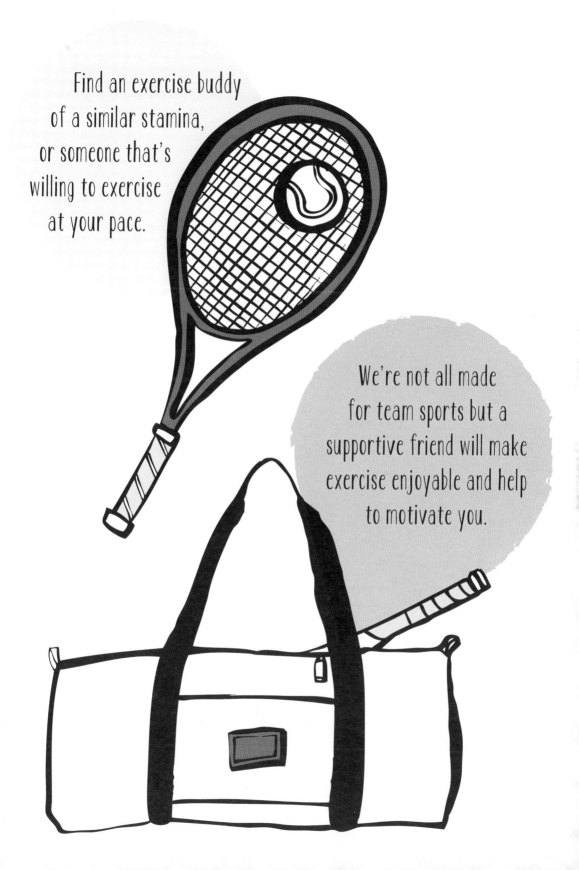

Monday

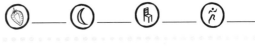

Tuesday

Wednesday

Thursday

Friday

🍓 —— 🌙 —— 🪑 —— 🏃 ——   🍓 —— 🌙 —— 🪑 —— 🏃 ——

Saturday

Sunday

🍓 —— 🌙 —— 🪑 —— 🏃 ——   🍓 —— 🌙 ——

🪑 —— 🏃 ——

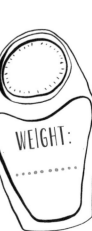

WEIGHT:

· · · · · · · · ·

BE AWARE

OF HOW MANY
CALORIES YOUR

DRINKS
CONTAIN

AS WELL AS
YOUR FOOD.

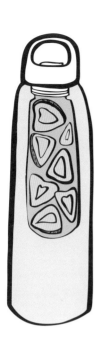

FILL THIS PAGE
WITH HEALTHY
ALTERNATIVE
DRINK RECIPES

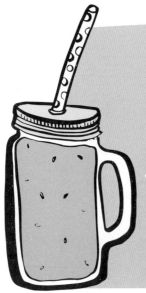

TURBO RECHARGER

This smoothie includes everything you need to revitalize your body after a strenuous training session: rehydrating melon, energy-boosting banana, vitamin C-packed grapes and iron-rich watercress – you're sorted!

Ingredients

¼ honeydew melon, peeled, deseeded and roughly chopped

1 banana, peeled and roughly chopped

1 kiwi fruit, peeled and roughly chopped

115 g/4 oz seedless green grapes

small handful of watercress (optional)

125 ml/4 fl oz unsweetened rice, almond or soya milk

small handful of crushed ice (optional)

Instructions

1. Put the melon, banana, kiwi fruit, grapes and watercress (if using) in a blender and whizz.

2. Add the milk and crushed ice (if using) and whizz again, until smooth.

3. Pour into a glass and serve immediately.

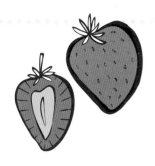
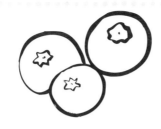
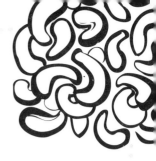

'Superfoods' have been called such because they are nutrient-dense ingredients with essential vitamins, minerals and antioxidants. It's worth noting these superfoods and thinking about how you can introduce them into your diet.

- Green vegetables such as spinach, kale and broccoli.

- Red berries such as strawberries and raspberries.

- Red vegetables such as peppers and beetroot.

- Orange fruit and vegetables such as sweet potato, carrots, mango and apricots.

- Fibre-rich fruit such as apples and pears.

- Probiotic yogurt, low-fat versions.

- Oily fish such as salmon, mackerel and sardines.

- Wholegrains such as brown rice and bread.

- Power pulses such as beans and lentils.

- Nuts, seeds and dates.

- Potassium fruits such as bananas and avocados.

- Plain chocolate.

- Green tea.

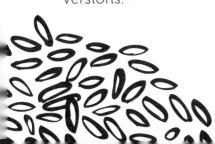

Monday

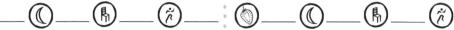

Tuesday

Wednesday

Thursday

🍓 ___ 🌙 ___ 🪑 ___ 🏃 ___

Friday

🍓 ___ 🌙 ___ 🪑 ___ 🏃 ___

Saturday

🍓 ___ 🌙 ___ 🪑 ___ 🏃 ___

Sunday

🍓 ___ 🌙 ___

🪑 ___ 🏃 ___

WEIGHT:

. . . .

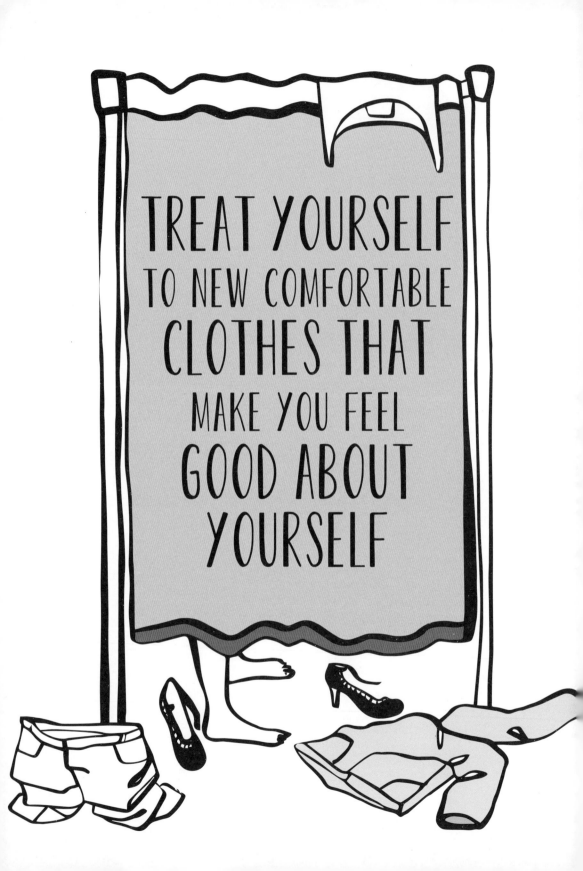

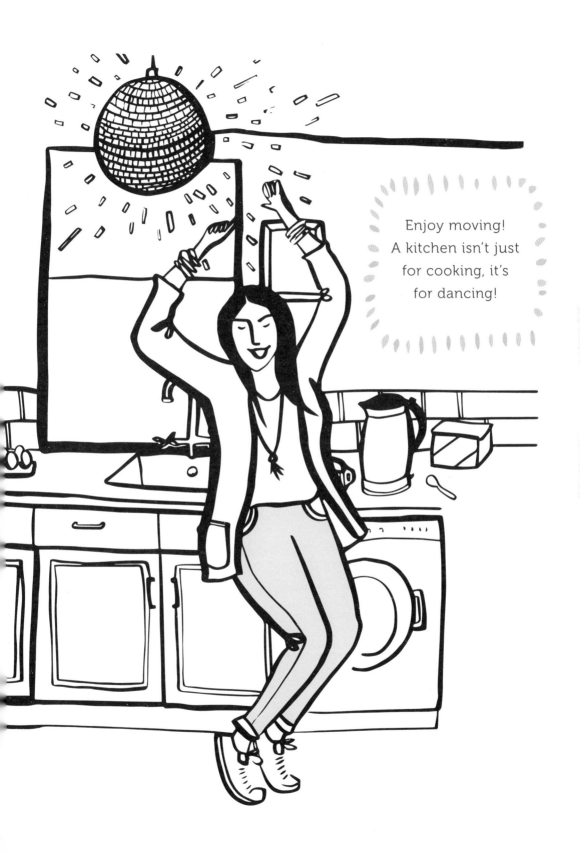

Enjoy moving!
A kitchen isn't just
for cooking, it's
for dancing!

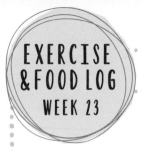

EXERCISE & FOOD LOG
WEEK 23

Monday

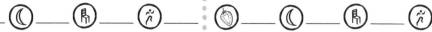

Tuesday

Wednesday

 —— —— —— ——

 —— —— —— ——

Thursday

🍓___ 🌙___ 🪑___ 🏃___

Friday

🍓___ 🌙___ 🪑___ 🏃___

Saturday

🍓___ 🌙___ 🪑___ 🏃___

Sunday

🍓___ 🌙___
🪑___ 🏃___

WEIGHT:

. . . .

Add some more tasty, yet healthy, recipes here.

EXERCISE & FOOD LOG
WEEK 24

Monday

🍓 —— ☾ —— 🪑 —— 🏃 ——

Tuesday

Wednesday

🍓 —— ☾ —— 🪑 —— 🏃 ——

🍓 —— ☾ —— 🪑 —— 🏃 ——

Thursday

🍓 ⃝___ ☾___ 🏃___ 🏃___

Friday

🍓 ⃝___ ☾___ 🏃___ 🏃___

Saturday

🍓 ⃝___ ☾___ 🏃___ 🏃___

Sunday

🍓 ⃝___ ☾___

🏃___ 🏃___

WEIGHT:

. . . .

Create balance in your life with these six things...

HEALTHY DIET

FRESH AIR

EXERCISE

SUNSHINE

WATER

REST

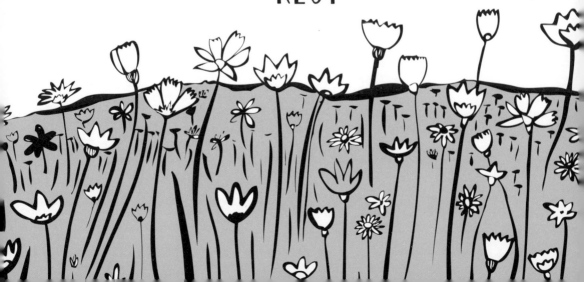

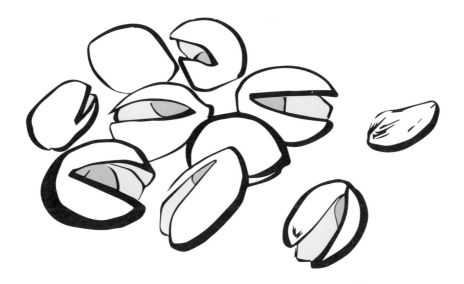

TAKE ADVANTAGE OF THE
PISTACHIO EFFECT

Shelling nuts, such as pistachios, or unwrapping
food can cut your calorie intake dramatically. The
empty shells or wrappers work as a visual reminder
of how much you've eaten.

Monday

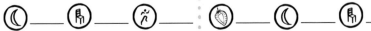

Tuesday

Wednesday

Thursday

Friday

Saturday

Sunday

WEIGHT:

....

WEEK 25 REFLECTION

Use this space to reflect on the past five weeks. Add doodles, progress graphs, lists, mood charts. Release your creativity.

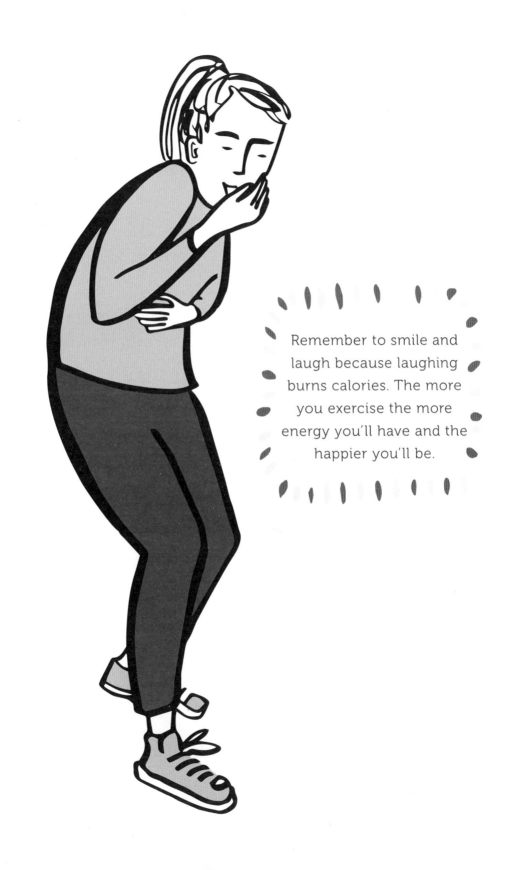

Remember to smile and laugh because laughing burns calories. The more you exercise the more energy you'll have and the happier you'll be.

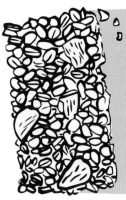

CHEWY APRICOT
& ALMOND ENERGY BARS

These energy bars are full of fruit and fibre and a first-rate choice for a portable, healthy mid-morning snack.

Ingredients

115 g/4 oz coconut oil

85 g/3 oz light muscovado sugar

60 g/2¼ oz almond butter, or other nut butter

1 dessert apple, cored and roughly grated

150 g/5½ oz porridge oats

40 g/1½ oz brown ground rice

55 g/2 oz unblanched almonds, roughly chopped

40 g/1½ oz sunflower seeds

200 g/7 oz dried apricots, diced

Instructions

1. Preheat the oven to 180°C/350°F/Gas Mark 4. Line a 20-cm/8-inch shallow square cake tin with non-stick baking paper.

2. Heat the oil and sugar in a medium-sized saucepan over a low heat until the oil has melted and the sugar is dissolved. Remove from the heat and stir in the almond butter. Add the apple, oats, ground rice, almonds and sunflower seeds, and mix together well.

3. Spoon two-thirds of the mixture into the prepared tin and press down firmly. Sprinkle over the apricots and press firmly into the base layer, then dot the remaining oat mixture over the top in a thin layer.

4. Bake in the oven for about 25 minutes, until the top is golden brown. Remove from the oven and leave to cool in the tin, then cut into 15 small rectangles. Store in the refrigerator for up to 3 days.

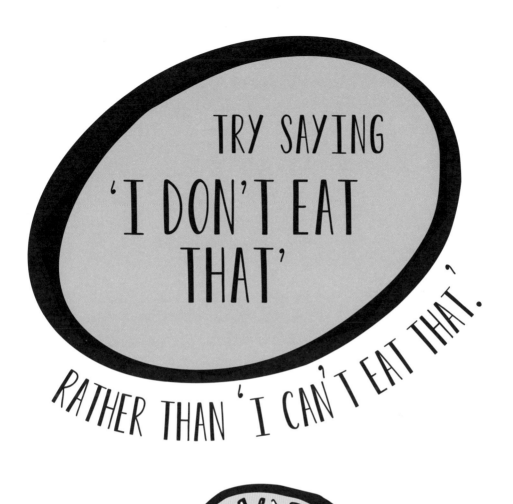

TRY SAYING 'I DON'T EAT THAT' RATHER THAN 'I CAN'T EAT THAT.'

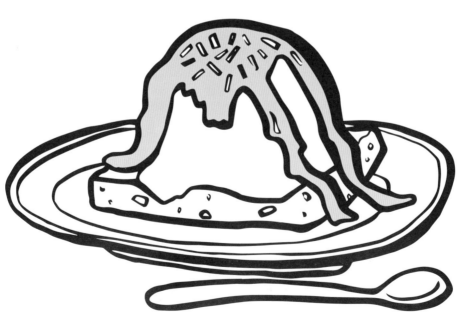

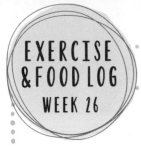

Monday

Tuesday

Wednesday

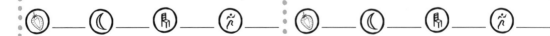

Thursday

🍓 ___ ☾ ___ 🪑 ___ 🏃 ___

Friday

🍓 ___ ☾ ___ 🪑 ___ 🏃 ___

Saturday

🍓 ___ ☾ ___ 🪑 ___ 🏃 ___

Sunday

🍓 ___ ☾ ___

🪑 ___ 🏃 ___

WEIGHT:

TAKE THE STAIRS NOT THE LIFT

A flight of stairs could be just the exercise you need on a busy day. Try this simple workout to get the heart pumping.

Get the blood flowing by running up the stairs and then walking down sideways. Do this five times leading with a different leg each time on the way down.

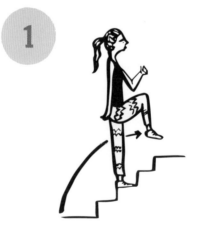

1

Stand at the bottom of the stairs, place your right foot on the second step then lift your left knee to your chest before quickly replacing your foot. Do this ten times on one side and then ten times on the other side.

2

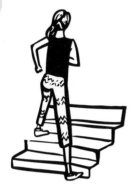 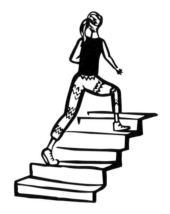

Walk up the stairs with your feet on the far edge of each
step to use the maximum width of the staircase, run down.
Do this five times.

3

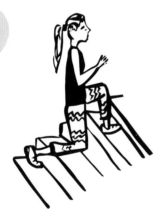

Take the stairs two at a time,
slowly with a deep lunge on
each step.

4

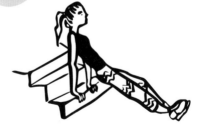

Finish with some tricep dips at
the bottom of the stairs.

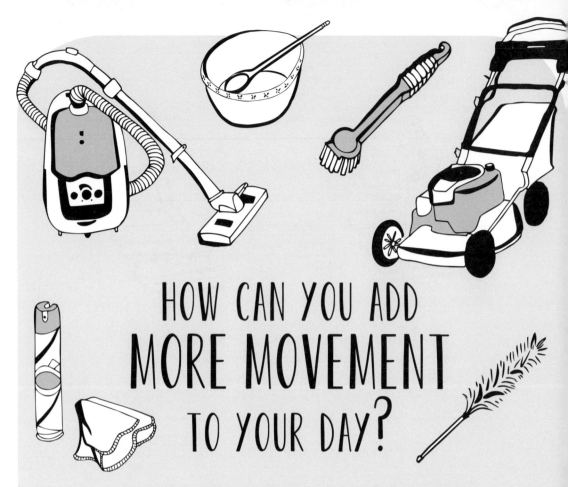

HOW CAN YOU ADD
MORE MOVEMENT
TO YOUR DAY?

If you don't have time to go to the gym or struggle
with certain types of exercises, think outside the box:
work your triceps by lifting a can up and down behind
your head ten times before making dinner. Star jumps
while you wait for the vegetables to boil.
Vacuum with added va-va-voom.

Write some inventive ways to add more movement to your life below.

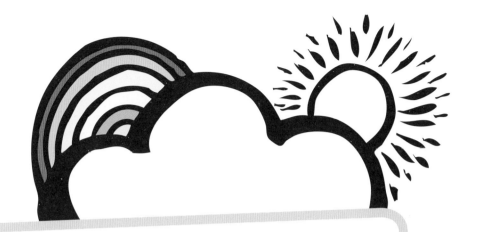

Breathing exercises can help you feel relaxed and are simple to do anywhere for five minutes. They're also great before bed if you have trouble sleeping.

Breathe in through your nose for two seconds and breathe out through pursed lips. Repeat ten times.

Then breathe in through your nose for four seconds and breathe out through pursed lips for four seconds. Repeat ten times.

As you get stronger you may want to increase to six and then eight seconds.

EXERCISE & FOOD LOG
WEEK 27

Monday

Tuesday

Wednesday

 — — —

 —

Thursday

🍓 —— ☾ —— 🪑 —— 🏃 ——

Friday

🍓 —— ☾ —— 🪑 —— 🏃 ——

Saturday

🍓 —— ☾ —— 🪑 —— 🏃 ——

Sunday

🍓 —— ☾ ——
🪑 —— 🏃 ——

WEIGHT:

. . . .

Find ways to feel good without using food. You don't necessarily have to spend money – take a long indulgent bath, play a board game with friends, ask someone to give you a massage, sing along to your favourite song, climb a big hill and take in the view, watch the sunrise...

Write a list of your own ideas here and then try one out.

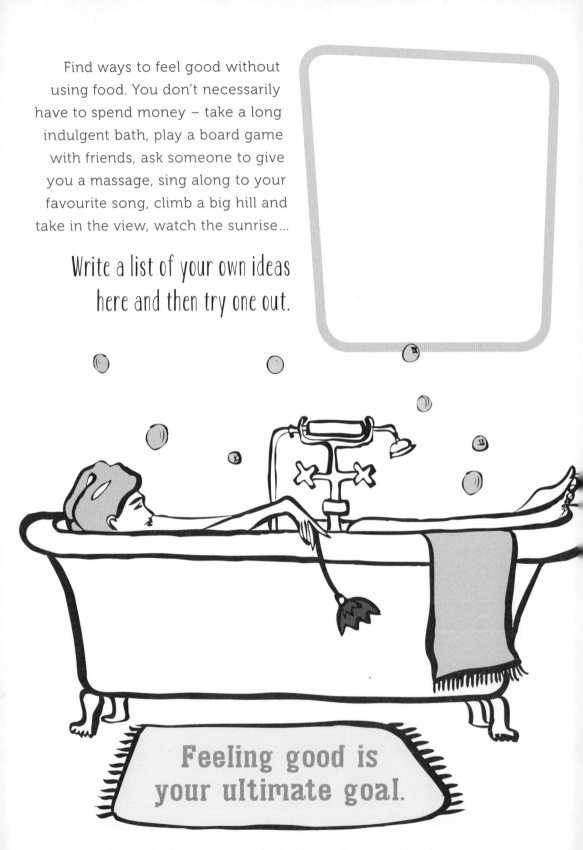

Feeling good is your ultimate goal.

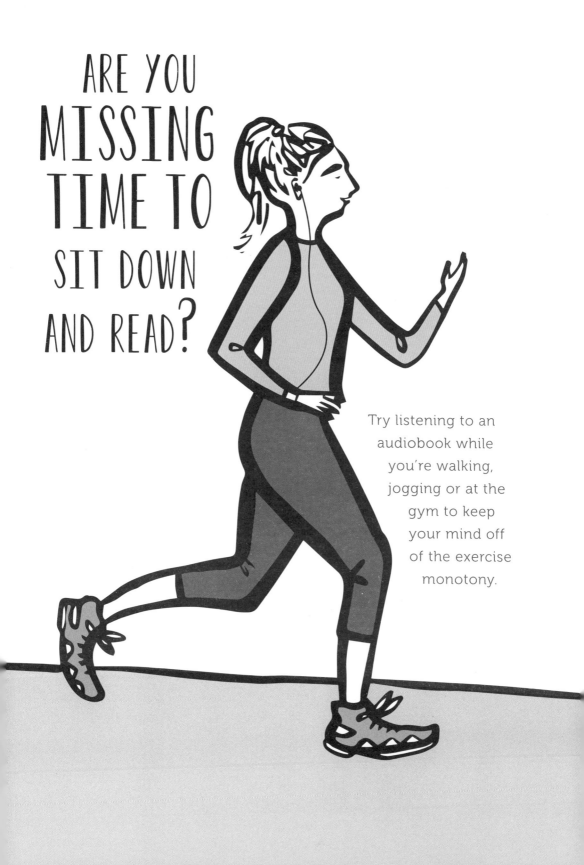

ARE YOU MISSING TIME TO SIT DOWN AND READ?

Try listening to an audiobook while you're walking, jogging or at the gym to keep your mind off of the exercise monotony.

EXERCISE & FOOD LOG
WEEK 28

Monday

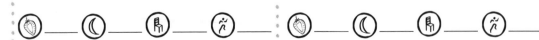

Tuesday

Wednesday

Thursday

Friday

🍓＿＿ 🌙＿＿ 🏋＿＿ 🏃＿＿

🍓＿＿ 🌙＿＿ 🏋＿＿ 🏃＿＿

Saturday

Sunday

🍓＿＿ 🌙＿＿ 🏋＿＿ 🏃＿＿

🍓＿＿ 🌙＿＿

🏋＿＿ 🏃＿＿

WEIGHT:

. . . .

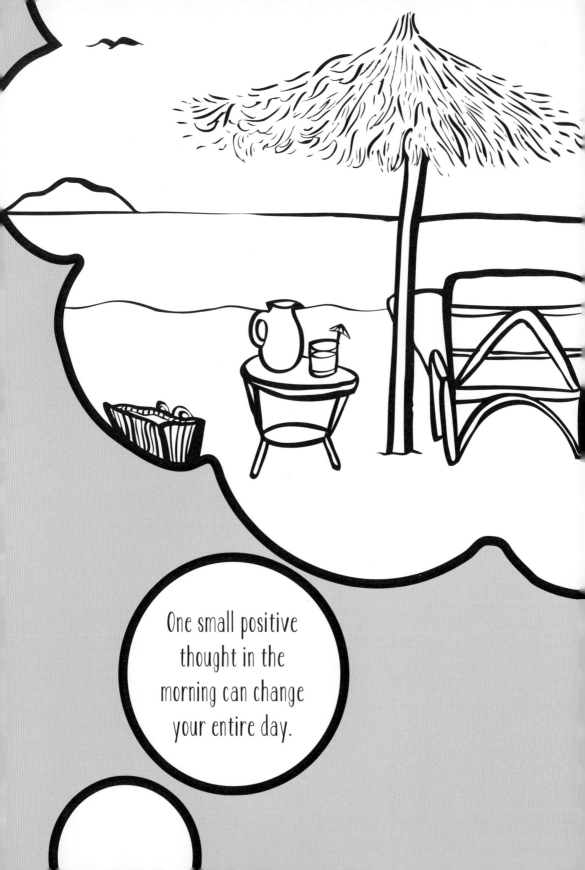

One small positive thought in the morning can change your entire day.

Try and give compliments to different people as often as you can to spread positivity.

Below, write five compliments you've been given that made you smile.

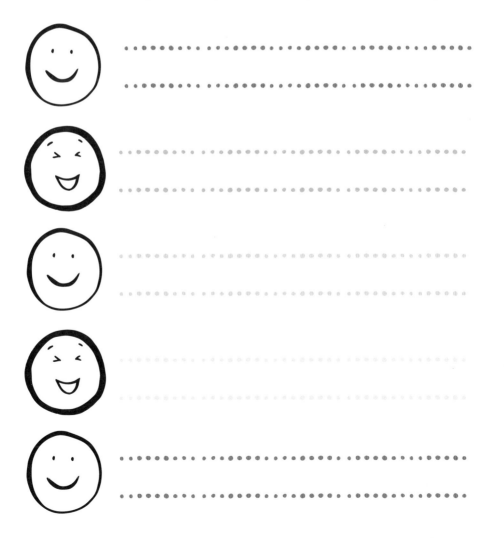

Monday

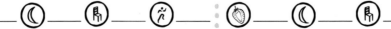

Tuesday

Wednesday

Thursday

🍓 ___ 🌙 ___ 🪑 ___ 🏃 ___

Friday

🍓 ___ 🌙 ___ 🪑 ___ 🏃 ___

Saturday

🍓 ___ 🌙 ___ 🪑 ___ 🏃 ___

Sunday

🍓 ___ 🌙 ___

🪑 ___ 🏃 ___

WEIGHT:

. . . .

Don't miss your friend's birthday meal because you're on a diet.

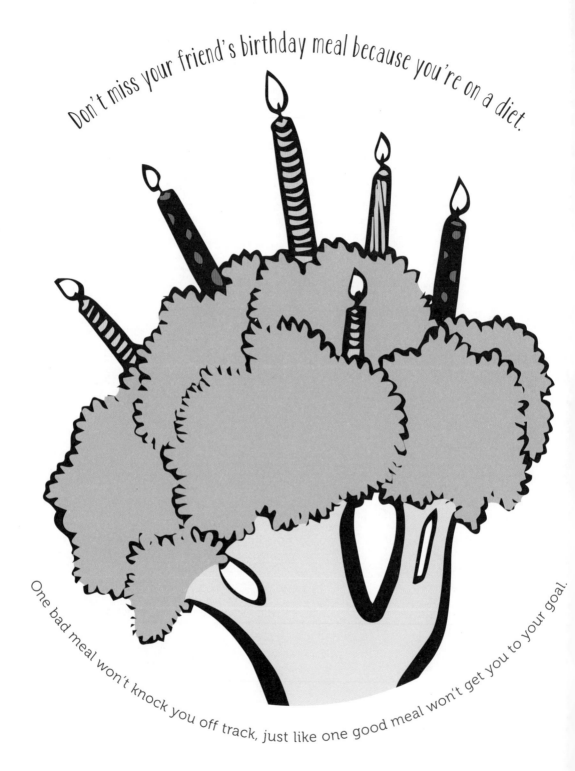

One bad meal won't knock you off track, just like one good meal won't get you to your goal.

FROM JUNK FOOD TO JOY FOOD

If you don't like it, don't eat it. The key is to make delicious food that happens to be healthy.

If you hate Zumba, don't go. Find foods and exercises that you genuinely enjoy and you might find it easier to stick with them.

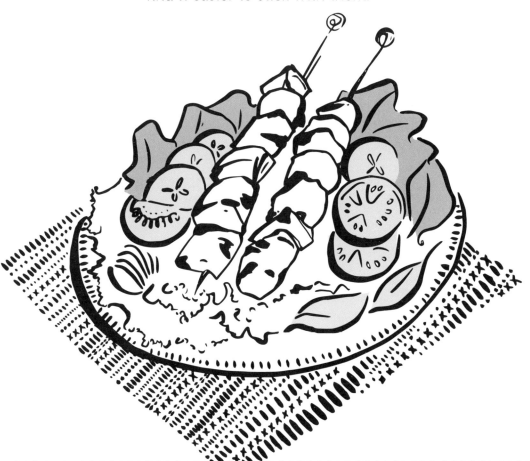

Monday

 — — —

Tuesday

Wednesday

 — — —

 — — —

Thursday

🍓 — 🌙 — 🪑 — 🏃 —

Friday

🍓 — 🌙 — 🪑 — 🏃 —

Saturday

🍓 — 🌙 — 🪑 — 🏃 —

Sunday

🍓 — 🌙 —
🪑 — 🏃 —

WEIGHT:
. . . .

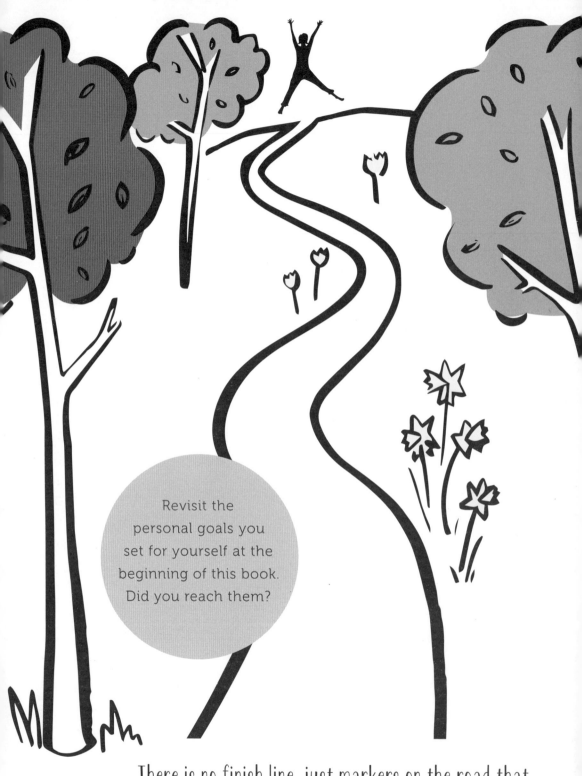

Revisit the personal goals you set for yourself at the beginning of this book. Did you reach them?

There is no finish line, just markers on the road that show us how far we've come and where we want to go.

A RECORD OF
WHERE YOU ARE NOW

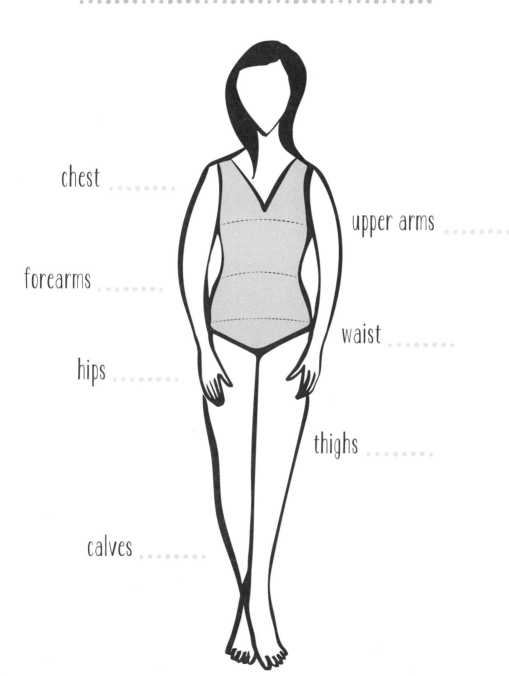

chest · · · · · · · · ·

upper arms · · · · · · · ·

forearms · · · · · · · ·

waist · · · · · · · ·

hips · · · · · · · ·

thighs · · · · · · · ·

calves · · · · · · · ·

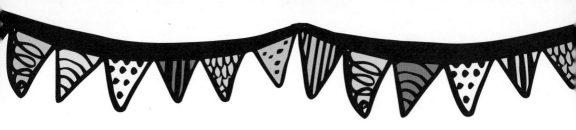

CONGRATULATIONS!

But this is not the end.

Use this journal to see how far
you've come, and then plan
the next steps to continue your
new healthy lifestyle.

Congratulate yourself for
achieving 30 weeks!

Repeat this mantra,

'BE POSITIVE, PATIENT AND PERSISTENT'.

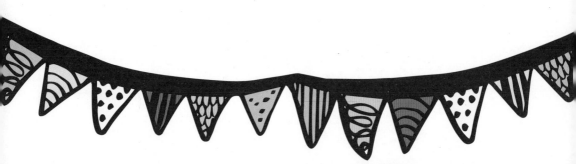